Animal Science: Sustenance, Conservation and Welfare of Animals

Edited by **Ryan Webber**

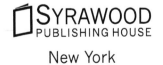

SYRAWOOD
PUBLISHING HOUSE

New York

Published by Syrawood Publishing House,
750 Third Avenue, 9th Floor,
New York, NY 10017, USA
www.syrawoodpublishinghouse.com

Animal Science: Sustenance, Conservation and Welfare of Animals
Edited by Ryan Webber

© 2016 Syrawood Publishing House

International Standard Book Number: 978-1-68286-004-5 (Hardback)

Contents

Preface

This book was inspired by the evolution of our times; to answer the curiosity of inquisitive minds. Many developments have occurred across the globe in the recent past which has transformed the progress in the field.

Animal science and welfare is rapidly expanding at a global scale. Scientists and researchers all over the world are devising new methods to better understand the physiology, genetics and behavior of animals. The chapters included herein bring forth some of the most innovative concepts and elucidate the unexplored aspects of animal science. The significance of animals for ecological sustainability, protection of endangered species, taxonomy and biodiversity of animals are some of the topics that have been discussed within this book. The extensive content of this book provides the readers with a thorough understanding of animal welfare. Students, researchers, experts and all associated with zoology and veterinary science will benefit alike from this book.

This book was developed from a mere concept to drafts to chapters and finally compiled together as a complete text to benefit the readers across all nations. To ensure the quality of the content we instilled two significant steps in our procedure. The first was to appoint an editorial team that would verify the data and statistics provided in the book and also select the most appropriate and valuable contributions from the plentiful contributions we received from authors worldwide. The next step was to appoint an expert of the topic as the Editor-in-Chief, who would head the project and finally make the necessary amendments and modifications to make the text reader-friendly. I was then commissioned to examine all the material to present the topics in the most comprehensible and productive format.

I would like to take this opportunity to thank all the contributing authors who were supportive enough to contribute their time and knowledge to this project. I also wish to convey my regards to my family who have been extremely supportive during the entire project.

Editor

Potential of Biological Processes to Eliminate Antibiotics in Livestock Manure: An Overview

Daniel I. Massé *, Noori M. Cata Saady and Yan Gilbert

Dairy and Swine Research and Development Centre, Agriculture and Agri-Food Canada, Sherbrooke, Quebec, J1M 0C8, Canada; E-Mail: Noori.saady@agr.gc.ca (N.M.C.S.); gilbertyan@hotmail.com (Y.G.)

* Author to whom correspondence should be addressed; E-Mail: daniel.masse@agr.gc.ca.

Simple Summary: Beside their use to treat infections, antibiotics are used excessively as growth promoting factors in livestock industry. Animals discharge in their feces and urine between 70%–90% of the antibiotic administrated unchanged or in active metabolites. Because livestock manure is re-applied to land as a fertilizer, concerns are growing over spread of antibiotics in water and soil. Development of antibiotic resistant bacteria is a major risk. This paper reviewed the potential of anaerobic digestion to degrade antibiotics in livestock manure. Anaerobic digestion can degrade manure-laden antibiotic to various extents depending on the concentration and class of antibiotic, bioreactor operating conditions, type of feedstock and inoculum sources.

Abstract: Degrading antibiotics discharged in the livestock manure in a well-controlled bioprocess contributes to a more sustainable and environment-friendly livestock breeding. Although most antibiotics remain stable during manure storage, anaerobic digestion can degrade and remove them to various extents depending on the concentration and class of antibiotic, bioreactor operating conditions, type of feedstock and inoculum sources. Generally, antibiotics are degraded during composting > anaerobic digestion > manure storage > soil. Manure matrix variation influences extraction, quantification, and degradation of antibiotics, but it has not been well investigated. Fractioning of manure-laden antibiotics into liquid and solid phases and its effects on their anaerobic degradation and the contribution of abiotic (physical and chemical) *versus* biotic degradation mechanisms need to be quantified for various manures, antibiotics types, reactor designs and temperature of operations.

More research is required to determine the kinetics of antibiotics' metabolites degradation during anaerobic digestion. Further investigations are required to assess the degradation of antibiotics during psychrophilic anaerobic digestion.

Keywords: antibiotics; livestock; manure; degradation; fate; anaerobic digestion

1. Introduction

Feeding antimicrobials (antibiotics) as growth promoter at sub-therapeutic doses to swine, cattle, poultry, and fish [1,2] is an integral part of the farm animal/fish production. Antibiotics are relatively recalcitrant to degradation. At significant concentrations, they impose bactericidal or antimicrobial effects which inhibit bacterial activity or growth. Animals excrete a significant fraction of antibiotics in feces and urine; therefore, there is substantial risk that unaltered or still active metabolites would be found in the environment. Different pathways for antibiotics introduction into the environment within an agricultural context were suggested [3]. Land application of livestock manure spreads antibiotics into environment at large scale. The excretion of wastes by grazing animals, atmospheric dispersal of feed and manure dust containing antibiotics [4] and the incidental release of products from spills or discharge are also potential pathways introducing antibiotics into the environment. Antibiotics in food products from animals and plants [5], the development and spread of antibiotic resistant bacteria [6], and the aquatic environments contamination from manure land application are concerns about agricultural antibiotic usage.

1.1. Antibiotic Consumption in Livestock Industry

Antibiotic consumption in livestock industry in USA, European countries and China is given in Figure 1. Notice that in the USA, for example, the quantity of antibiotics used in 2004 is 108 times that used in 1950. This is partially because the recommended levels of growth-promoting antibiotics in poultry and pig diets increased from 4 ppm for the narrow spectrum and 10 ppm for the broad-spectrum antibiotics in 1950s to 200 ppm nowadays. About 91% of livestock operations in the USA use 11.2 million kg antibiotics sold over-the-counter as growth promoters annually [6–10]. Antibiotics fed to animals end up in manure and eventually in the environment.

Figure1. Quantities of antibiotics consumed by livestock in animal feed (Data from [7–9,11]).

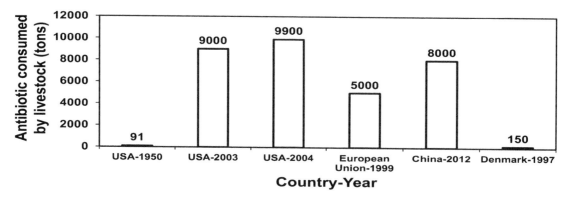

1.2. Types of Antibiotics Used in Livestock

Major antibiotics used in livestock: Various antibiotics classes are used to various extents and frequencies therapeutically and sub-therapeutically in livestock industry [2] including:

1. b-Lactams: *penicillins*: amoxicillin, ampicillin, benzylpenicillin, cloxacilin, dicloxacilin, flucloxacillin, methicillin, mezlocillin, nafcillin, oxacillin, piperacillin, phenoxymethylcillin.
2. Macrolides: azithromycin, clarithromycin, clindamycin, *erythromycin*, roxithromycin, spiramycin, *tylosin*, vancomycin.
3. Sulphonamides: *sulphadimidine, sulphamethoxazole*.
4. *Trimethoprim*.
5. Fluorochinolones: ciprofloxacin, ofloxacin.
6. *Tetracyclines: chlortetracycline, doxycycline, oxytetracycline, tetracycline*.
7. Polyether antibiotic: *monensin*

The antibiotics in Italic font are the major antibiotics usually used in swine and cattle while other antibiotics are less frequent. Pan *et al.* [12] reported detection frequencies of 85%–97% (tetracyclines), 52% (sulphonamides), and 5% (macrolide) in 126 swine manure samples collected from 21 animal feeding operation in Shandong-China. Similar results were reported in China (Chen *et al.* [11] and Japan [13]). Tetracyclines (especially oxytetracycline (OTC) and chlortetracycline (CTC)) occur worldwide in lagoon samples or manures from livestock husbandry [14–18].

1.3. Excretion of Antibiotics in Livestock Manure

Animals excrete significant proportion of antibiotics (17%–90% for livestock) [7,19–21] directly into urine and feces, unchanged or as active metabolites (epimers or isomers) of the parent species [22]. Table 1 gives the percentage of antibiotics excreted by animals with their metabolic status (changed or unchanged from their administrated form). Some metabolites are more potent than their parent compounds, while others such as acetic conjugates of sulphonamides can revert back to their parent compounds during manure storage [23].

Table 1. Level of excretion of antibiotics from animals.

Antibiotic	Source of manure	Excretion level (%)	Status	Reference
Chlortetracycline	Steers feces	75	Not reported	[24]
Tetracycline	Animal feces	25	Not reported	[25]
Tylosin	Urine	50–60	Unchanged	[25]
Oxytetracycline	Castrate sheeps	21	Unchanged	[26]
Chlortetracycline	Young bulls	17–75	Unchanged	[26]
Tylosin	Pigs	40	Unaltered or as potent metabolites	[27]
Monensin	Beef cattle feces	40%	Unchanged	[28]
Virginiamycin	Piggeries liquid manure	20	After several days of storage	[29]
Oxytetracycline	Calves manure (feces, urine, and bedding)	23	Not reported	[30]

1.4. Concentration of Antibiotics in Livestock Manure

Typically, antibiotic concentrations in manure are between 1 to 10 mg·kg^{-1} or L^{-1} but may reach levels $\geq$ 200 mg·kg^{-1} or L^{-1} [20]. Concentrations of 100's mg·kg^{-1} or mg·L^{-1} of veterinary antibiotics have been found in animal excreta in China [11,31,32]. It is not clear whether the high variation in the detected concentrations and the antibiotics excretion by animals were due to individual differences regarding antibiotics metabolism or to an inadequate extraction and quantification methods used during these studies. The concentration of the most commonly used antibiotics have been reported to be as high as 216 mg·L^{-1} of swine, beef, and poultry/turkey manures [21].

Several studies have confirmed that antibiotics used in animal production are present in fresh manure, manure storage tanks, soil, surface and underground water [33,34]. Jacobsen and Halling-Sørensen [18] detected tetracycline and sulphonamides in swine manure, but no tylosin was detected because of poor recoveries of tylosin from manure. De Liguoro et al. [35] found 0.11 mg·kg^{-1} of tylosin and 10 mg·kg^{-1} of OTC in fresh calf manure, but found negligible concentrations of these compounds in soil and water. Dolliver and Gupta [36] found that 1.2% to 1.8% chlortetracycline, monensin and tylosin were lost from manure stockpile by runoff water. Campagnolo et al. [37] found significant quantity of macrolides, sulphonamides and fluoroquinolones in the nearby surface water.

While the measured concentrations shown in Table 2 and elsewhere assess for the presence of antibiotics in various environmental samples and collectively provided strong evidences of their widespread in manure, each study reports its own quantification technique with particular recovery efficiencies, sensibility and reliability.

Table 2. Concentration of some antibiotics in manures.

Antibiotic	Matrix	Concentration	Reference
Oxytetracycline	Manure	136 mg·L^{-1}	[14]
Chlortetracycline		46 mg·L^{-1}	
Tetracycline	Swine manure	98 mg·L^{-1}	
Oxytetracycline		354 mg·L^{-1}	
Chlortetracycline		139 mg·L^{-1}	[11]
Doxycycline		37 mg·L^{-1}	
Sulfadiazine		7.1 mg·L^{-1}	
Tetracycline	Swine manure	30 mg·kg^{-1} DM	[18]
Sulphonamides		2 mg·kg^{-1} DM	
Tylosin	Fresh calf manure	0.11 mg·kg^{-1}	[35]
Oxytetracycline		10 mg·kg^{-1}	
Chlortetracycline,	Beef manure stockpile	6.6 mg·kg^{-1}	
Monensin		120 mg·kg^{-1}	[36]
Tylosin		8.1 mg·kg^{-1}	
Oxytetracycline	Cow manure	0.5–200 mg·L^{-1}	[38]
Chlortetracycline	Swine manure	764.4 mg·L^{-1}	[12]
Chlortetracycline	Swine manure storage	1 mg·L^{-1}	[37]
Oxytetracycline	lagoon	0.41 mg·L^{-1}	

There is no standardized and reliable method for antibiotics quantification in complex matrices, such as soil and biological sludge, making inter- and even intra-study comparisons difficult. Most studies report results without sufficiently describing the condition of the manure handling and management before sampling. Partitioning of antibiotics into the liquid and solid phases affects the results. For example, sampling a leaching manure pile would indicate the solid phase fraction of the antibiotics rather than the total concentration.

Most of the antibiotic residues in manure form complexes with soluble organics and remain stable during manure storage. When manure is applied to agriculture fields, a fraction of the antibiotics becomes mobile with the flow of water in the soil and contaminate the surrounding environment including surface and groundwater. The extent of fractioning of an antibiotic between solid and aqueous phases, and hence its mobility, depends on the properties of the antibiotic, soil, and the hydrological effects. More research is required to understand kinetics of biodegradation and potencies of degraded products of various antibiotics in different environments (soils, manures and waste water).

1.5. Environmental Transport of Antibiotics from Livestock Manure

Antibiotics behavior and transport in the environment are related to their physicochemical properties [33]. Numerous antibiotics comprise a non-polar core associated with polar functional moieties; many antibiotics are amphiphilic or amphoteric and ionized. However, physicochemical properties vary widely among compounds from the various structural classes and antibiotics of the same class do not necessarily exhibit identical behaviors. Adsorption of antibiotics to the organic and mineral exchange sites in soil is mostly due to charge transfer and ion interaction and not only to hydrophobic partitioning [34].

Wu *et al.* [39] demonstrated that ciprofloxacin, tetracycline, doxycycline, and clindamycin were strongly sorbed on aerobically digested biosolids, while sulfamethazine and sulfamethoxazole were only weakly sorbed to particles. Davis *et al.* [40] investigated the transport of seven different antibiotics used in animal production during a simulated rainfall event and determined their association with the sediment or the aqueous phase. They reported that the percentage of partitioning of the antibiotics into (aqueous, solid) phases for sulfathiazole (77,23), sulfamethazine (95,5), monensin (91,9), erythromycin (26,74), and tylosin (23,77). Therefore, sulfathiazole, sulfamethazine, and monensin mostly associated with aqueous phase while tylosin and erythromycin associated with the solid phase. The tendency of some antibiotics to adsorb on particles reduces their bioavailability [39,41] and results in low degradation rates. Chen *et al.* [11] found tetracycline, oxytetracycline, chlortetracycline, and doxycycline (0.1–205 µg·kg^{-1}) in manure-amended soils near swine farms. Dolliver *et al.* [5] found that corn, lettuce, and potato took sulfamethazine from a manure-amended soil and accumulated 0.1 mg to 1.2 mg sulfamethazine kg^{-1} of dry plant tissue after 45 days of growth; although the accumulated concentration is relatively low it might still pose a health concern. Therefore, surface waters, agricultural soils, and groundwaters may become reservoirs to antibiotics because of the current manure management practices [42,43]. Many antibiotics have short half-lives (days to weeks) [41,44], but at high concentration some persist for months to years within agricultural-related matrices [27,45]. For example, manure storage does not affect tetracyclines and sulfadiazine [11]. Lamshöft *et al.* [46] observed that metabolites of sulfadiazine have been reversibly converted to sulfadiazine; therefore, they suggested that frequent fertilization of soil by manure contaminated with sulfadiazine and its metabolites may cause them to accumulate in soil and results in environmental contamination. The physicochemical properties, the structure of antibiotics and their degradation by-products determine whether they degrade during biological treatment [47], some compounds and their metabolites may persist for days to months [11].

Evaluating the data available on degradation and fate of antibiotics during anaerobic digestion of livestock manure is essential to the development of this technology as an integral part of the strategy to control the spread of antibiotic resistant bacteria. This paper summarizes what is currently known about behavior, of the major antibiotic used in livestock therapeutically or as growth promoters, during anaerobic digestion, their metabolic by-products, and fractioning into aqueous and solid fractions. There is little information regarding the effect and fate (removal) of antibiotics during the anaerobic digestion of manure [30,48].

2. Persistence and Biodegradation of Antibiotics during Biological Processes of Manure Treatment

2.1. Persistence of Antibiotics in Manure

A summary of the reported half-life ($t_{1/2}$) of some antibiotics during manure storage or in soil environment is given in Table 3. Generally, a wide range of half-lives has been reported in the scientific literature regarding antibiotic degradation from different environmental conditions.

Table 3. Half life of antibiotics under storage and natural environment conditions.

Antibiotic	Medium matrix	Half-life (days unless indicated otherwise)	Reference
Tetracycline	Biosolids storage	37 to >77	[49]
Tetracycline	Stored feedlot manure	17.2	[50]
Chlortetracycline	Composted manure	3	[51]
Chlortetracycline	Dairy manure	6.8	[50]
Chlortetracycline	Stored feedlot manure	13.5	[50]
Oxytetracycline	Stockpiled fresh manure (low-intensity composting)	21	[35]
Oxytetracycline	Dairy manure	17.7	[50]
Oxytetracycline	Stored feedlot manure	31.1	[50]
Oxytetracycline	Horse manure	8.4	[50]
Tylosin	Aerobic soil-manure slurry	3.3–8.1	[41]
Olaquindox	Aerobic soil-manure slurry	5.8–8.8	[41]
Metronidazole	Aerobic soil-manure slurry	13.1–26.9	[41]
Erythromycin	Storage of pig manure	41	[52]
Erythromycin	Biosolids storage	7.0–17	[49]
Roxithromycin	Storage of pig manure	130	[52]
Salinomycin	Storage of pig manure	6	[52]
Doxycycline	Biosolids storage	53 to >77	[49]
Clindamycin	Biosolids storage	1.0–1.6	[49]
Clarithromycin	Biosolids storage	1.1–1.9	[49]

Storteboom *et al.* [50] found that OTC persists in dairy manure ($t_{1/2}$ = 17.7 d) longer than in horse manure ($t_{1/2}$ = 8.4 d). However, matrix differences could have influenced antibiotic recoveries during extraction and quantification methods used and thus biased half-lives.

In addition, different types of biological processes affect antibiotic persistence differently; for example, chlortetracycline half-life has been found to increase in the order: composting > manure storage > soil. Half-lives for the primary degradation in aerobic soil-manure slurries ranging from 3.3 to 8.1 days for tylosin, 5.8 to 8.8 days for olaquindox, and 13.1 to 26.9 days for metronidazole were observed [41]. Schlüsener *et al.* [53] indicated that erythromycin, roxithromycin and salinomycin, tetracycline, doxycycline, clindamycin, and clarithromycin were more persistent under anaerobic conditions than aerobic condition with a longer $t_{1/2}$ by a factor of 1.5 to 2, suggesting that aerobic degradation might be a more important mechanism to eliminate these compounds from the environment [49]. However, the results were not sufficiently strong to support this assumption. The authors emphasized on the need to obtain more data for compounds from different classes to support this assumption and to perform further research to clarify the degradation pathways and identify the metabolites. Also, the poor antibiotic recoveries related to the extraction techniques used (31%–83% recoveries) and high matrix effects (50%–90%) can account in part for the variation in results. Table 4 gives the half-lives of major antibiotic classes in manure environment; notice that tetracyclines and quinolones are very persistent with an average half-live of around 100 days. Recently, improved extraction, cleaning, and quantification methods have been developed. Hence, better recoveries are expected from recent studies on antibiotics degradation during the anaerobic digestion of manure.

Table 4. Persistence of major classes of veterinary antibiotics in manure (adapted from Boxall *et al.* [3]).

Chemical group	Half-life (d)	Persistence class
Aminoglycosides	30	Moderately persistent
β-lactams	5	Slightly persistent
Macrolides	<2 to 21	Impersistent to slightly persistent
Quinolones	100	Very persistent
Sulphonamides	<8 to 30	Slightly to moderately persistent
Tetracyclines	100	Very persistent

2.2. Biodegradation Level of Antibiotics in Manure Biological Treatment

Bioavailability of antibiotics determines their degradation rate, however, bioavailability depends on the compound's hydrophobicity [54]. Therefore, antibiotic's chemical properties and manure-related matrix characteristics modify the antibiotics' reluctance to biodegradation and play a significant role in antibiotic removal, respectively [50]. Motoyama *et al.* [13] related differences in the measured concentrations of the same antibiotic in different types of manures (swine, cattle, and horses) to the specific adsorption characteristics of the different manures' matrices. The physicochemical characteristics of various antibiotics correlated with their degradation profiles and support these assumptions [34].

Degradation of antibiotics in compost, soil, manure, and sediments follows the same metabolic mechanisms [55] though differences among different media matrices affect the fractioning of antibiotics between liquid and solid phases. Results of antibiotics' degradation studies should be considered cautiously depending on how the bioassay has been conducted, the extraction recovery efficiency, and the resolution of the quantification protocol. Studies reporting on degradation of antibiotics as sole substrate using a standardized bacterial consortium in closed bottles incubated in the dark at 20 °C and assessing the oxygen consumed on theoretical oxygen demand (ThOD) [56] provide a limited information. More reliable results should be obtained from studies conducted with antibiotic-containing manure simulating real situations using mixed anaerobic cultures and monitored by gas production, COD removal, and VFAs consumption. Table 5 presents a summary of antibiotics degradation in livestock manure biological treatment. Notice that the removal of oxytetracycline varied from as low as 55%–70% (soil) to 55%–75% (anaerobic digestion) to 85%–99% (composting). Except for the 99% removal during composting, all other removals efficiencies have been achieved using the same initial oxytetracycline concentration (20 mg·L^{-1}).

Careful examination of Table 5 reveals several trends. The high removals during composting are likely due to the effects of the additional aerobic bioactivity compared to anaerobic digestion alone. Although both soil and composting share the same aerobic-anoxic conditions composting showed higher removals likely because of the presence of good inoculum compared to soil condition. No sound conclusion could be drawn regarding the effect of the biological action temperature on antibiotic removal. For example, mesophilic and thermophilic anaerobic digestion operation showed higher removals of chlortetracycline than psychrophilic operation, however, for monensin both psychrophilic and mesophilic showed low removals compared to thermophilic. Interestingly, oxytetracycline was removed in soil by almost the same efficiency at 5 °C and 15 °C, while at 25 °C a 20% increase in the removal efficiency was observed.

Although the degradation half-lives were reported for antibiotics in stored solids or in soil where there is a "passive" biodegradation, these values do not reflect degradation rates in the presence of an active biomass such as in waste treatment processes. Aerobic and anaerobic waste treatment processes have shown their efficiency to remove many xenobiotics and pharmaceuticals from effluents. Some studies have evaluated the biodegradability, mostly in aerobic conditions, of various antibiotics used for human health and animal production. Al-Ahmad et al. [57] have shown, when testing the biodegradability of cefotiam, ciprofloxacin, meropenem, penicillin G, and sulfamethoxazole using closed bottle test [56], that only pencillin G was biodegradable to some degree (27%), prolonging the test from 28 to 40 days increased the removal to 35%. Using the same test to evaluate the biodegradability of ciproflaxin, ofloxacin and metronidazole, Kümmerer et al. [58] observed no biodegradation of those antibiotics, without loss of their genotoxicity.

Wang et al. [59] found that degradation kinetics of sulfadimethoxine was affected by its initial concentration because microorganisms are inhibited at high antibiotic concentrations; this result could presumably be extrapolated to any antimicrobials degradation kinetic. Shi et al. [60] found that tetracycline and sulfamethoxydiazine initial concentrations of up to 50 mg·L^{-1} decreased by 50% within 12 h of continuous anaerobic digestion (OLR 1.88 kg COD m^{-3}·d^{-1}) and only traces of antibiotics were detected after 2–3 days. These researchers did not provide evidence whether the reduction of the antibiotics concentration was due to sorption or biodegradation. Loke et al. [61] found a half-life value lower than 2 days for tylosin A in manure spiked with 25 mg·L^{-1} during anaerobic digestion of swine waste at 20 °C. Moreover, in aerobic conditions the disappearance rates of tylosin A increased with increasing concentrations of solids, but it was not clear if removal was due to bacterial or abiotic degradation, or that sorption on manure particles was responsible for low aqueous antibiotic concentrations. Loke *et al.* [61] did not observe instant sorption of tylosin on manure particles, with 102% to 108% recoveries during method validation. However, recovery efficiencies were not assessed for long term contact between the antibiotic and manure particles. Hence, it is plausible that the more concentrated solids adsorb more of the antibiotic over time and less is recovered, which gives the impression that the half-life is shorter in this condition.

Table 5. Biodegradation of antibiotics in manure.

Treatment	Antibiotic	Concentration	Observed reduction	Reference
I. Anaerobic digestion				
Anaerobic digestion of swine manure 21 days	Chlortetracycline	6.5 mg·L^{-1} 8.3 mg·L^{-1} 5.9 mg·L^{-1}	7% (22 °C) 80% (38 °C) 98% (55 °C)	[62]
Anaerobic digestion of cattle manure (28 days)	Monensin	0.74 mg·L^{-1} 0.36 mg·L^{-1} 0.30 mg·L^{-1}	3% (22 °C) 8% (38 °C) 27% (55 °C)	[62]
Batch anaerobic digestion	Oxytetracycline	20 mg·L^{-1}	55%–73% at 37 °C	[63]
Anaerobic sequence batch reactor (ASBR)	Tylosin A	1.6 mg·kg^{-1} 5.8 mg·kg^{-1}	Degraded to <detection limit. Decreased to 0.01 mg·L^{-1} in 48 h	[1]
Swine manure from lagoons	Tylosin	0–400 mg·kg^{-1}	95%–75%	[64]
II. Composting				
Composting (22–35 days)	Chlortetracycline	1.5 mg·kg^{-1}	99%	[65]
	Monensin Tylosin	11.9 mg·kg^{-1} 3.7 mg·kg^{-1}	54%	[65]
	Sulfamethazine	10.8 mg·kg^{-1}	–76%	[65]
Composting beef manure (35 days) abiotic removal	Oxytetracycline	115 µg·g^{-1} DM	99% (laboratory) 25% (22 °C)	[51]
Composting	Oxytetracycline Tetracycline Chlortetracycline Levofloxacine Ciprofloxacine Erythromycin Sulfamonomethoxine Sulfamethoxazole Trimethoprim Carbamazepine	20 mg·L^{-1}	85% 92% 90% (all removals 81% at 38 °C) 100% 67% 79% 95% 86% 37%	[13]
III. Manure amended soil				
Soil	Tetracycline Chlortetracycline	5–300 µg·kg^{-1} 4.7 µg·kg^{-1}	0% 0%	[66]
	Sulphanilamide	0.25–1.0 mg·L^{-1}	0%	[67]
	Tylosin	5.6 µg·L^{-1}	0%	[68]
	Erythromecin	5.6 µg·L^{-1}	25%	[68]
Storage	Sulfadiazine Difloxacin	156 mg·L^{-1} 17.6 mg·L^{-1}	0% (10 °C and 20 °C) 7% (10 °C and 20 °C)	[46]

The effects of individual and mixtures of antimicrobials on manure biological treatment depend on inhibition and resistance mechanisms, the manure matrix, the composition of the microbial community, biotic and abiotic degradation of antimicrobials, and sorption of antimicrobials [69].

2.2.1. Tetracyclines

Abiotic mechanisms were responsible for a removal of 98% of CTC (initial concentration $(C_i) = 113$ $\mu g \cdot g^{-1}$) during 30 days of beef manure composting (TS = 30%) [9]. However, there was an increased loss of extractable CTC residues with increased time, probably due to sorption to organic matter, rendering its quantification difficult. Approximately 60% removal of OTC ($C_i = 9.8$ $mg \cdot L^{-1}$) was achieved in 64 days by anaerobic digestion at 35 °C (TS 4.0% to 4.7%) yielding a calculated half-life of 56 days for OTC [30,48]. Also, approximately 75% removal of buffer extractable CTC ($C_i = 5.9$ $mg \cdot L^{-1}$) was achieved in 33 days by anaerobic digestion at 35 °C yielding a calculated value half-life of about 18 days. However, these removals during anaerobic digestion cannot be directly related to biological activity or abiotic mechanisms since no sorption analysis was performed. Anaerobic digestion decreased concentrations of OTC from 13.5, 56.9 and 95.0 $mg \cdot L^{-1}$ to 5.7, 26.6 and 30.7 $mg \cdot L^{-1}$ in 21 days, respectively, while CTC was decreased from 9.8, 46.1 and 74.0 $mg \cdot L^{-1}$ to 0.9, 4.0 and 7.5 $mg \cdot L^{-1}$, respectively [70]. CTC was transformed and epimerized at faster rates than that for OTC. CTC decreased in the solid fraction at a slower rate than that observed in the aqueous phase likely because water-extractable antibiotics are most "available" for degradation by microorganisms and that 100% of CTC concentration has been found water-extractable [65]. Finally, the degradation product and epimer of CTC, 4-epi-chlortetracycline (ECTC), was completely removed at high rate [70]. Arikan et al. [48] and [30] reported a significant removal of the parent compounds of CTC and OTC during the first 10 days of incubation, then, OTC was degraded in 60–70 days whereas CTC was removed at a slower rate. These finding agrees with the half-life of OTC (22–27 days) determined during batch anaerobic digestion of manure [63].

The adsorption of OTC and CTC was limited by the available superficial area of the inoculum and pig manure [70]. Furthermore, OTC and CTC form strong complexes with divalent cations, which are abundant in pig manure, adsorb onto proteins, particles and organic matter [71]. At 35 °C and pH 7, 40% and 60% of OTC and CTC, respectively, were removed in the first hour. 4-epi-oxytetracycline (EOTC), an epimer of OTC and ECTC degraded quickly. After 7 days, 6% of the initial amount of OTC remained in the assay [70].

Álvarez et al. [70] determined also the first-order degradation constants for OTC (0.045 to 0.058 d^{-1}) and CTC (0.169 to 0.216 d^{-1}) while Arikan et al. [30] reported lower first-order degradation constants (0.012 and 0.039 d^{-1} for OTC and CTC, respectively). This inconsistency might have been caused by the higher organic matter content in the assays (50 $g \cdot L^{-1}$ of cattle manure), which could have increased the stability of both compounds due to their strong adsorption onto the solid fraction [70].

The half-life of oxytracycline in manure was 30 days and it was detectable (820 $ug \cdot kg^{-1}$) after 5 months of maturation [35]. Søeborg et al. [72] suggested that some portion of chlortetracycline degradation during composting may be due to abiotic processes.

2.2.2. Tylosin

De Liguoro *et al.* [35] found that tylosin degraded rapidly and it was undetectable in manure after 45 days; no trace (>10 ug·L^{-1}) of the compound was detected in soil or surrounding water. Chelliapan *et al.* [64] reported that 95% tylosin reduction with a COD reduction of 93% were achieved in an up-flow anaerobic stage reactor (UASR) treating pharmaceutical wastewater (contains tylosin 0 to 400 mg·L^{-1}) at a HRT of 4 d and OLR of 1.86 kg COD m^{-3}·d^{-1}. However, at concentrations of 600 and 800 mg·L^{-1} the COD reduction was 85% and the tylosin removal was 75% [64]. They concluded that tylosin concentrations ≤ 400 mg·L^{-1} had a minimal effect on reactor performance. Methanogens were active in the reactor even at 800 mg·L^{-1} tylosin which did not affect the CH$_4$ yield. Similar findings that such as high concentrations of tylosin are unlikely to create problems in the treatment of wastewater by anaerobic digestion have been reported in other studies [73,74].

The tylosin A half-life of (2.5 h) in high-rate anaerobic digester is shorter than its half-lives (2–8 days) in soils or passively stored manure [1,41,61,75]. Tylosin was degraded in soil columns (half-life 3.3–8.1 days) [41]. Kolz *et al.* [27] found that 90% of tylosin A in anaerobic sludge was sorbed and degraded (abiotic or biotic) within 5 days in anaerobic digestion. Angenent *et al.* [1] concluded that tylosin was removed by degradation rather than sorption in anaerobic batch experiment and ASBR; with dehydroxy-tylonolide as a by-product. Such conclusion could be explained by the fact that water-extractable antibiotics are most "available" for degradation by microorganisms given that 85% of the total-extractable concentration of tylosin was water-extractable [65].

Chelliapan *et al.* [76] reported tylosin (initial concentration 10–220 mg·L^{-1}) removal of 70–88% in upflow anaerobic stage reactor operating at OLR 1.86 kg COD m^{-3}·d^{-1} with a COD removal of 70%–75%. At higher OLR (2.84–3.73 kg COD m^{-3}·d^{-1}), tylosin removal increased and was stable between 93%–99% despite that the COD removal declined to about 45%. Obviously, there is no agreement on which mechanism is responsible for the removal of tylosin in anaerobic digestion.

2.2.3. Other Antibiotics

Sulfamethazole was utilized as carbon and nitrogen source by the microorganisms in absence of those nutrients, but remained intact in the presence of acetate and ammonium [77]. Antibiotics like ciprofloxacin, ofloxacin, and virginiamycin degrade very slowly and may persist in soil in its original form up to 30–80 days while bambermycin and erythromycin completely degrade in a period of one month at temperatures ranging from 20–30 °C [21].

Carballa *et al.* [78] found that mesophilic anaerobic digestion (STR of 30 days) degraded 99 and 94% of sulfamethoxazole, and roxithromycin, respectively. Water-extractable antibiotics are most "available" for degradation by microorganisms. The percentage of initial water-extractable antibiotic concentration out of the total-extractable was 40% for monensinand 85% for sulfamethazine [65].

Kim *et al.* [79] observed decrease in tetracyclines, sulfamethazine, and tylosin concentrations from 20 mg·kg^{-1} to less than 0.8, 0.2, and 1.0 mg·kg^{-1}, respectively, during composting of pig manure with saw dust. Presence of saw dust correlated with the decline in tetracyclines and sulfamethazine concentrations, but not with tylosin. Again, it is debatable to compare results from different studies because of the utilization of various antibiotic quantification techniques having different reliabilities and precision. Moreover, most of these studies did not discuss the possibility that antibiotics would be adsorbed on particles and thus not quantified, biasing the degradation rates obtained.

2.4. Metabolites

Fedler and Day [80] suggested that the antibiotics themselves may not inhibit bacteria but their metabolites produced in the gastrointestinal tract of the animal may. 4-Epi-oxytetracycline (EOTC), a-apo-oxytetracycline (a-Apo-OTC) and b-apo-oxytetracycline (b-Apo-OTC) are degradation products of oxytetracycline (OTC) [48] whereas 4-epi-chlortetracycline (ECTC) is a degradation product and epimer of chlortetracycline (CTC). These metabolites are similar to their parent in creating complexes with metal ions, humic acids, proteins, particles and organic matter in the manure matrix [71] thus they are strongly adsorbed in manure. Unfortunately, almost all of the studies on antibiotics in manure focused on the parent compounds except several studies on OTC and CTC where antibiotic degradation progenies were monitored. It has been concluded that antibiotic metabolites produced in the gastrointestinal tract of the animal may inhibit bacterial activity more than the original molecule [73]. On the contrary, Halling-Sørensen *et al.* [81] found that the degradation products of OTC have less biological activity on sludge and soil bacteria than OTC. These authors also found a similar trend of biotransformation between the parent and the intermediate compounds (EOTC and ECTC), as well as the removal of these intermediates [70].

3. Required Future Research

Developing standard protocols to assess the impact, degradation, and fate of various antibiotics and their metabolites during anaerobic digestion is essential to enable a reasonable comparison among results generated from different studies. Assessing the effect of culture matrices, solid content, and nature of manure organic fraction on the degradation dynamic of various antibiotic during anaerobic digestion is required with a focus on kinetic and metabolic modeling and simulation of inhibition, recovery, and adaptation mechanisms. Particularly, better understanding and prediction of the contribution of abiotic (physical and chemical) *versus* biotic degradation mechanisms of the different antibiotic classes is required. Fractioning of manure-laden antibiotics into liquid and solid phases and its effects on their anaerobic degradation needs to be understood and quantified under various manure classes, antibiotics types, reactor design and operation. For design purposes, kinetic data is required for the degradation of the antibiotic parent compounds and their metabolites in different anaerobic reactor designs and operation. Effects of process staging and modification need to be explored to avoid operational problems due to the effects of high antibiotics' concentrations on the anaerobic digestion. Potential of psychrophilic anaerobic digestion of livestock manure to eliminate antibiotics and antibiotic resistant bacteria has not been investigated yet.

4. Conclusions

Most antibiotics form complexes with metals and soluble organics in manure and remain stable during storage, however; anaerobic digestion can degrade them to various extents depending on the concentration and class of antibiotic, operation condition, and type of culture.

Antibiotic's chemical properties and manure-related matrix characteristics interact to modify their reluctance to biodegradation and play a significant role in antibiotics' removal. The physicochemical characteristics of various antibiotics correlate with their degradation profile. Antibiotics' degradation during anaerobic digestion depends on their water-extractability which affects their bioavailability to microorganisms. Therefore, fractioning of antibiotics into liquid and solid phases of manure, its effects on their anaerobic degradation, and contribution of abiotic (physical and chemical) *versus* biotic degradation mechanisms need to be determined and quantified for various manures, antibiotics types, reactor designs and operation conditions. Different types of biological processes affect antibiotic persistence differently; composting > anaerobic digestion > soil.

Antibiotics and their metabolites are strongly adsorbed in manure because of chemical combination with metals and organics. More research is required to evaluate kinetics and fate of antibiotic degradation progenies. It is strongly suggested that standard analytical protocols be developed for the detection, extraction, and quantification antibiotics from manure. Such standard methods will enable sound comparison of the results generated from different studies and making better conclusion regarding the impact, degradation, and fate of various antibiotics and their metabolites during anaerobic digestion. Assessing the effect of culture matrices, solid content, and nature of manure organic fraction on the degradation kinetics of various antibiotics during anaerobic digestion is required with a focus on kinetic, metabolic modeling, simulation of inhibition, recovery, and adaptation mechanisms. Further investigations are required to assess the degradation of antibiotics during psychrophilic anaerobic digestion.

Acknowledgments

This project has been financially supported through contributions from Agriculture and Agri-Food Canada, the Canadian Dairy Commission and Dairy Farmers of Canada under the Dairy Research Cluster Program.

Author Contributions

Conceived the project on antibiotic degradation: DIM; obtained the financial support: DIM; performed the critical literature review: IG, DIM and NMCS; wrote the paper: IG, DIM and NMCS.

Conflicts of Interest

The authors declare no conflict of interest.

References

1. Angenent, L.T.; Mau, M.; George, U.; Zahn, J.A.; Raskin, L. Effect of the presence of the antimicrobial tylosin in swine waste on anaerobic treatment. *Water Res.* **2008**, *42*, 2377–2384.

2. Kemper, N.; Färber, H.; Skutlarek, D.; Krieter, J. Analysis of antibiotic residues in liquid manure and leachate of dairy farms in northern germany. *Agr. Water Manag.* **2008**, *95*, 1288–1292.

3. Boxall, A.B.A.; Fogg, L.A.; Blackwell, P.A.; Blackwell, P.; Kay, P.; Pemberton, E.J.; Croxford, A. Veterinary medicines in the environment. *Rev. Environ. Contam. Toxicol.* **2004**, *180*, 1–91.

4. Hamscher, G.; Pawelzick, H.; Sczesny, S.; Nau, H.; Hartung, J. Antibiotics in dust originating from a pig-fattening farm: A new source of health hazard for farmers? *Environ. Health Perspect.* **2003**, *111*, 1590–1594.

5. Dolliver, H.; Kumar, K.; Gupta, S. Sulfamethazine uptake by plants from manure-amended soil. *J. Environ. Qual.* **2007**, *36*, 1224–1230.

6. Mellon, M.; Benbrook, C.; Benbrook, K. *Hogging it: Estimates of Antimicrobial Abuse in Livestock*; Union of Concerned Scientists: Cambridge, MA, USA, 2001.

7. Sarmah, A.K.; Meyer, M.T.; Boxall, A.B.A. A global perspective on the use, sales, exposure pathways, occurrence, fate and effects of veterinary antibiotics (VAs) in the environment. *Chemosphere* **2006**, *65*, 725–759.

8. Shea, K.M. Antibiotic resistance: What is the impact of agricultural uses of antibiotics on children's health? *Pediatrics* **2003**, *112*, 253–258.

9. Arikan, O.A.; Mulbry, W.; Rice, C. Management of antibiotic residues from agricultural sources: Use of composting to reduce chlortetracycline residues in beef manure from treated animals. *J. Hazard. Mater.* **2009**, *164*, 483–489.

10. National Research Council. *The Use of Drugs in Food Animals: Benefits and Risks*; National Academy Press: Washington, DC, USA, 1999; p. 25.

11. Chen, Y.; Zhang, H.; Luo, Y.; Song, J. Occurrence and assessment of veterinary antibiotics in swine manures: A case study in east china. *Chin. Sci. Bull.* **2012**, *57*, 606–614.

12. Pan, X.; Qiang, Z.; Ben, W.; Chen, M. Residual veterinary antibiotics in swine manure from concentrated animal feeding operations in shandong province, china. *Chemosphere* **2011**, *84*, 695–700.

13. Motoyama, M.; Nakagawa, S.; Tanoue, R.; Sato, Y.; Nomiyama, K.; Shinohara, R. Residues of pharmaceutical products in recycled organic manure produced from sewage sludge and solid waste from livestock and relationship to their fermentation level. *Chemosphere* **2011**, *84*, 432–438.

14. Martínez-Carballo, E.; González-Barreiro, C.; Scharf, S.; Gans, O. Environmental monitoring study of selected veterinary antibiotics in animal manure and soils in austria. *Environ. Pollut.* **2007**, *148*, 570–579.

15. Aust, M.O.; Godlinski, F.; Travis, G.R.; Hao, X.; McAllister, T.A.; Leinweber, P.; Thiele-Bruhn, S. Distribution of sulfamethazine, chlortetracycline and tylosin in manure and soil of canadian feedlots after subtherapeutic use in cattle. *Environ. Pollut.* **2008**, *156*, 1243–1251.

16. Christian, T.; Schneider, R.J.; Färber, H.A.; Skutlarek, D.; Meyer, M.T.; Goldbach, H.E. Determination of antibiotic residues in manure, soil, and surface waters. *Acta Hydrochim. Hydrobiol.* **2003**, *31*, 36–44.

17. Karci, A.; Balcioğlu, I.A. Investigation of the tetracycline, sulfonamide, and fluoroquinolone antimicrobial compounds in animal manure and agricultural soils in turkey. *Sci. Total Environ.* **2009**, *407*, 4652–4664.

18. Jacobsen, A.M.; Halling-Sørensen, B. Multi-component analysis of tetracyclines, sulfonamides and tylosin in swine manure by liquid chromatography-tandem mass spectrometry. *Anal. Bioanal. Chem.* **2006**, *384*, 1164–1174.

19. Bound, J.P.; Voulvoulis, N. Pharmaceuticals in the aquatic environment—A comparison of risk assessment strategies. *Chemosphere* **2004**, *56*, 1143–1155.

20. Kumar, K.; Gupta, S.C.; Chander, Y.; Singh, A.K. Antibiotic use in agriculture and its impact on the terrestrial environment. *Adv. Agron.* **2005**, *87*, 1–54.

21. *Antibiotics in Manure and Soil—A Grave Threat to Human and Animal Health*; Policy Paper 43; National Academy of Agriculture Science: New Delhi, India, 2010; p. 20.

22. Mackie, R.I.; Koike, S.; Krapac, I.; Chee-Sanford, J.; Maxwell, S.; Aminov, R.I. Tetracycline residues and tetracycline resistance genes in groundwater impacted by swine production facilities. *Anim. Biotech.* **2006**, *17*, 157–176.

23. Boxall, A.B.; Blackwell, P.; Cavallo, R.; Kay, P.; Tolls, J. The sorption and transport of a sulphonamide antibiotic in soil systems. *Toxicol. Lett.* **2002**, *131*, 19–28.

24. Elmund, G.K.; Morrison, S.M.; Grant, D.W.; Nevins, M.P. Role of excreted chlortetracycline in modifying the decomposition process in feedlot waste. *Bull. Environ. Contam. Toxicol.* **1971**, *6*, 129–132.

25. Feinman, S.E.; Matheson, J.C. *Draft Environmental Impact Statement Subtherapeutic Antibacterial Agents in Animal Feeds*; FDA: Rockville, MD, USA, 1978.

26. Montforts, M.H.M.M.; Kalf, D.F.; Van Vlaardingen, P.L.A.; Linders, J.B.H.J. The exposure assessment for veterinary medicinal products. *Sci. Total Environ.* **1999**, *225*, 119–133.

27. Kolz, A.C.; Moorman, T.B.; Ong, S.K.; Scoggin, K.D.; Douglass, E.A. Degradation and metabolite production of tylosin in anaerobic and aerobic swine-manure lagoons. *Water Environ. Res.* **2005**, *77*, 49–56.

28. Donoho, A.; Manthey, J.; Occolowitz, J.; Zornes, L. Metabolism of monensin in the steer and rat. *J. Agr. Food Chem.* **1978**, *26*, 1090–1095.

29. Cocito, C. Antibiotics of the virginiamycin family, inhibitors which contain synergistic components. *Microbiol. Rev.* **1979**, *43*, 145–198.

30. Arikan, O.A. Degradation and metabolization of chlortetracycline during the anaerobic digestion of manure from medicated calves. *J. Hazard. Mater.* **2008**, *158*, 485–490.

31. Hu, X.G.; Luo, Y.; Zhou, Q.X.; Xu, L. Determination of thirteen antibiotics residues in manure by solid phase extraction and high performance liquid chromatography. *Chin. J. Anal. Chem.* **2008**, *36*, 1162–1166.

32. Xian, Q.; Hu, L.; Chen, H.; Chang, Z.; Zou, H. Removal of nutrients and veterinary antibiotics from swine wastewater by a constructed macrophyte floating bed system. *J. Environ. Manag.* **2010**, *91*, 2657–2661.

33. Pruden, A. Production and transport of antibiotics from cafos. In *Hormones and Pharmaceuticals Generated by Concentrated Animal Feeding Operations*; Springer-Verlag: New York, NY, USA, 2009; pp. 63–70.

34. Thiele-Bruhn, S. Pharmaceutical antibiotic compounds in soils—A review. *J. Plant Nutr. Soil Sci.* **2003**, *166*, 145–167.

35. De Liguoro, M.; Cibin, V.; Capolongo, F.; Halling-Sørensen, B.; Montesissa, C. Use of oxytetracycline and tylosin in intensive calf farming: Evaluation of transfer to manure and soil. *Chemosphere* **2003**, *52*, 203–212.

36. Dolliver, H.A.S.; Gupta, S.C. Antibiotic losses from unprotected manure stockpiles. *J. Environ. Qual.* **2008**, *37*, 1238–1244.

37. Campagnolo, E.R.; Johnson, K.R.; Karpati, A.; Rubin, C.S.; Kolpin, D.W.; Meyer, M.T.; Esteban, J.E.; Currier, R.W.; Smith, K.; Thu, K.M.; *et al.* Antimicrobial residues in animal waste and water resources proximal to large-scale swine and poultry feeding operations. *Sci. Total Environ.* **2002**, *299*, 89–95.

38. Ince, B.; Coban, H.; Turker, G.; Ertekin, E.; Ince, O. Effect of oxytetracycline on biogas production and active microbial populations during batch anaerobic digestion of cow manure. *Bioprocess Biosyst. Eng.* **2013**, *36*, 541–546.

39. Wu, C.; Spongberg, A.L.; Witter, J.D. Sorption and biodegradation of selected antibiotics in biosolids. *J. Environ. Sci. Health A* **2009**, *44*, 454–461.

40. Davis, J.G.; Truman, C.C.; Kim, S.C.; Ascough, J.C., II; Carlson, K. Antibiotic transport via runoff and soil loss. *J. Environ. Qual.* **2006**, *35*, 2250–2260.

41. Ingerslev, F.; Halling-Sørensen, B. Biodegradability of metronidazole, olaquindox, and tylosin and formation of tylosin degradation products in aerobic soil-manure slurries. *Ecotoxicol. Environ. Safety* **2001**, *48*, 311–320.

42. Hu, X.; Zhou, Q.; Luo, Y. Occurrence and source analysis of typical veterinary antibiotics in manure, soil, vegetables and groundwater from organic vegetable bases, northern china. *Environ. Pollut.* **2010**, *158*, 2992–2998.

43. Chang, X.; Meyer, M.T.; Liu, X.; Zhao, Q.; Chen, H.; Chen, J.A.; Qiu, Z.; Yang, L.; Cao, J.; Shu, W. Determination of antibiotics in sewage from hospitals, nursery and slaughter house, wastewater treatment plant and source water in chongqing region of three gorge reservoir in china. *Environ. Pollut.* **2010**, *158*, 1444–1450.

44. Teeter, J.S.; Meyerhoff, R.D. Aerobic degradation of tylosin in cattle, chicken, and swine excreta. *Environ. Res.* **2003**, *93*, 45–51.

45. Winckler, C.; Grafe, A. Use of veterinary drugs in intensive animal production: Evidence for persistence of tetracycline in pig slurry. *J. Soils Sediments* **2001**, *1*, 66–70.

46. Lamshöft, M.; Sukul, P.; Zuhlke, S.; Spiteller, M. Behaviour of (14)c-sulfadiazine and (14)c-difloxacin during manure storage. *Sci. Total Environ.* **2010**, *408*, 1563–1568.

47. Ben, W.; Qiang, Z.; Adams, C.; Zhang, H.; Chen, L. Simultaneous determination of sulfonamides, tetracyclines and tiamulin in swine wastewater by solid-phase extraction and liquid chromatography-mass spectrometry. *J. Chromatogr. A* **2008**, *1202*, 173–180.

48. Arikan, O.A.; Sikora, L.J.; Mulbry, W.; Khan, S.U.; Rice, C.; Foster, G.D. The fate and effect of oxytetracycline during the anaerobic digestion of manure from therapeutically treated calves. *Process Biochem.* **2006**, *41*, 1637–1643.

49. Wu, C.; Spongberg, A.L.; Witter, J.D. Determination of the persistence of pharmaceuticals in biosolids using liquid-chromatography tandem mass spectrometry. *Chemosphere* **2008**, *73*, 511–518.

50. Storteboom, H.N.; Kim, S.C.; Doesken, K.C.; Carlson, K.H.; Davis, J.G.; Pruden, A. Response of antibiotics and resistance genes to high-intensity and low-intensity manure management. *J. Environ. Qual.* **2007**, *36*, 1695–1703.

51. Arikan, O.A.; Sikora, L.J.; Mulbry, W.; Khan, S.U.; Foster, G.D. Composting rapidly reduces levels of extractable oxytetracycline in manure from therapeutically treated beef calves. *Bioresour. Technol.* **2007**, *98*, 169–176.

52. Schlusener, M.P.; Bester, K. Persistence of antibiotics such as macrolides, tiamulin and salinomycin in soil. *Environ. Pollut.* **2006**, *143*, 565–571.

53. Schlüsener, M.; von Arb, M.; Bester, K. Elimination of macrolides, tiamulin, and salinomycin during manure storage. *Arch. Environ. Contam. Toxicol.* **2006**, *51*, 21–28.

54. Ingerslev, F.; Halling-Sorensen, B. Biodegradability properties of sulfonamides in activated sludge. *Environ. Toxicol. Chem.* **2000**, *19*, 2467–2473.

55. Büyüksönmez, F.; Rynk, R.; Hess, T.F.; Bechinski, E. Occurrence, degradation and fate of pesticides during composting: Part II: Occurrence and fate of pesticides in compost and composting systems. *Compost Sci. Utilization* **2000**, *8*, 61–81.

56. 301D Closed Bottle Test. In *Guidelines for Testing of Chemicals*; Adopted by the Council on 17th July 1992; OECD: Paris, France, 1992.

57. Al-Ahmad, A.; Daschner, F.D.; Kümmerer, K. Biodegradability of cefotiam, ciprofloxacin, meropenem, penicillin g, and sulfamethoxazole and inhibition of waste water bacteria. *Arch. Environ. Contam. Toxicol.* **1999**, *37*, 158–163.

58. Kümmerer, K.; Al-Ahmad, A.; Mersch-Sundermann, V. Biodegradability of some antibiotics, elimination of the genotoxicity and affection of wastewater bacteria in a simple test. *Chemosphere* **2000**, *40*, 701–710.

59. Wang, Q.-Q.; Bradford, S.A.; Zheng, W.; Yates, S.R. Sulfadimethoxine degradation kinetics in manure as affected by initial concentration, moisture, and temperature. *J. Environ. Qual.* **2006**, *35*, 2162–2169.

60. Shi, J.C.; Liao, X.D.; Wu, Y.B.; Liang, J.B. Effect of antibiotics on methane arising from anaerobic digestion of pig manure. *Anim. Feed Sci. Technol.* **2011**, *166–167*, 457–463.

61. Loke, M.-L.; Ingerslev, F.; Halling-Sørensen, B.; Tjørnelund, J. Stability of tylosin a in manure containing test systems determined by high performance liquid chromatography. *Chemosphere* **2000**, *40*, 759–765.

62. Varel, V.H.; Wells, J.E.; Shelver, W.L.; Rice, C.P.; Armstrong, D.L.; Parker, D.B. Effect of anaerobic digestion temperature on odour, coliforms and chlortetracycline in swine manure or monensin in cattle manure. *J. Appl. Microbiol.* **2012**, *112*, 705–715.

63. Turker, G.; Ince, O.; Ertekin, E.; Akyol, C.; Ince, B. Changes in performance and active microbial communities due to single and multiple effects of mixing and solid content in anaerobic digestion process of otc medicated cattle manure. *Int. J. Renew. Energ. Res.* **2013**, *3*, 144–148.

64. Chelliapan, S.; Wilby, T.; Sallis, P.J. Performance of an up-flow anaerobic stage reactor (UASR) in the treatment of pharmaceutical wastewater containing macrolide antibiotics. *Water Res.* **2006**, *40*, 507–516.

65. Dolliver, H.; Gupta, S.; Noll, S. Antibiotic degradation during manure composting. *J. Environ. Qual.* **2008**, *37*, 1245–1253.

66. Hamscher, G.; Sczesny, S.; Hoper, H.; Nau, H. Determination of persistent tetracycline residues in soil fertilized with liquid manure by high-performance liquid chromatography with electrospray ionization tandem mass spectrometry. *Anal. Chem.* **2002**, *74*, 1509–1518.

67. Frankenberger, W.T.; Tabatabai, M.A. Transformations of amide nitrogen in soils1. *Soil Sci. Soc. Am. J.* **1982**, *46*, 280–284.

68. Gavalchin, J.; Katz, S.E. The persistence of fecal-borne antibiotics in soil. *J. AOAC Int.* **1994**, *77*, 481–485.

69. Amin, M.M.; Zilles, J.L.; Greiner, J.; Charbonneau, S.; Raskin, L.; Morgenroth, E. Influence of the antibiotic erythromycin on anaerobic treatment of a pharmaceutical wastewater. *Environ. Sci. Technol.* **2006**, *40*, 3971–3977.

70. Álvarez, J.A.; Otero, L.; Lema, J.M.; Omil, F. The effect and fate of antibiotics during the anaerobic digestion of pig manure. *Bioresource Technol.* **2010**, *101*, 8581–8586.

71. Loke, M.L.; Jespersen, S.; Vreeken, R.; Halling-Sørensen, B.; Tjørnelund, J. Determination of oxytetracycline and its degradation products by high-performance liquid chromatography-tandem mass spectrometry in manure-containing anaerobic test systems. *J. Chromatogr. B* **2003**, *783*, 11–23.

72. Søeborg, T.; Ingerslev, F.; Halling-Sørensen, B. Chemical stability of chlortetracycline and chlortetracycline degradation products and epimers in soil interstitial water. *Chemosphere* **2004**, *57*, 1515–1524.

73. Massé, D.I.; Lu, D.; Masse, L.; Droste, R.L. Effect of antibiotics on psychrophilic anaerobic digestion of swine manure slurry in sequencing batch reactors. *Bioresource Technol.* **2000**, *75*, 205–211.

74. Poels, J.; Van Assche, P.; Verstraete, W. Effects of disinfectants and antibiotics on the anaerobic digestion of piggery waste. *Agr. Wastes* **1984**, *9*, 239–247.

75. Rabølle, M.; Spliid, N.H. Sorption and mobility of metronidazole, olaquindox, oxytetracycline and tylosin in soil. *Chemosphere* **2000**, *40*, 715–722.

76. Chelliapan, S.; Wilby, T.; Sallis, P.J.; Yuzir, A. Tolerance of the antibiotic tylosin on treatment performance of an up-flow anaerobic stage reactor (UASR). *Water Sci. Technol.* **2011**, *63*, 1599–1606.

77. Drillia, P.; Dokianakis, S.N.; Fountoulakis, M.S.; Kornaros, M.; Stamatelatou, K.; Lyberatos, G. On the occasional biodegradation of pharmaceuticals in the activated sludge process: The example of the antibiotic sulfamethoxazole. *J. Hazard. Mater.* **2005**, *122*, 259–265.

78. Carballa, M.; Omil, F.; Ternes, T.; Lema, J.M. Fate of pharmaceutical and personal care products (ppcps) during anaerobic digestion of sewage sludge. *Water Res.* **2007**, *41*, 2139–2150.

79. Kim, K.R.; Owens, G.; Ok, Y.S.; Park, W.K.; Lee, D.B.; Kwon, S.I. Decline in extractable antibiotics in manure-based composts during composting. *Waste Manag.* **2012**, *32*, 110–116.

80. Fedler, C.B.; Day, D.L. Anaerobic Digestion of Swine Manure Containing an Antibiotic Inhibitor. *Trans. ASAE* **1985**, *28*, 523–530.

81. Halling-Sørensen, B.; Sengeløv, G.; Tjørnelund, J. Toxicity of tetracyclines and tetracycline degradation products to environmentally relevant bacteria, including selected tetracycline-resistant bacteria. *Arch. Environ. Contam. Toxicol.* **2002**, *42*, 263–271.

2

Emerging and Re-Emerging Zoonoses of Dogs and Cats

Bruno B. Chomel

Department of Population Health and Reproduction, School of Veterinary Medicine, University of California, Davis, CA 95616, USA; E-Mail: bbchomel@ucdavis.edu.

Simple Summary: Dogs and cats have been sharing our environment for a long time and as pets they bring major psychological well-being to our modern urbanized society. However, they still can be a source of human infection by various pathogens, including viruses, bacteria, parasites, and fungi.

Abstract: Since the middle of the 20th century, pets are more frequently considered as "family members" within households. However, cats and dogs still can be a source of human infection by various zoonotic pathogens. Among emerging or re-emerging zoonoses, viral diseases, such as rabies (mainly from dog pet trade or travel abroad), but also feline cowpox and newly recognized noroviruses or rotaviruses or influenza viruses can sicken our pets and be transmitted to humans. Bacterial zoonoses include bacteria transmitted by bites or scratches, such as pasteurellosis or cat scratch disease, leading to severe clinical manifestations in people because of their age or immune status and also because of our closeness, not to say intimacy, with our pets. Cutaneous contamination with methicillin-resistant *Staphylococcus aureus*, *Leptospira* spp., and/or aerosolization of bacteria causing tuberculosis or kennel cough are also emerging/re-emerging pathogens that can be transmitted by our pets, as well as gastro-intestinal pathogens such as *Salmonella* or *Campylobacter*. Parasitic and fungal pathogens, such as echinococcosis, leishmaniasis, onchocercosis, or sporotrichosis, are also re-emerging or emerging pet related zoonoses. Common sense and good personal and pet hygiene are the key elements to prevent such a risk of zoonotic infection.

Keywords: zoonoses; dog; cat; emerging diseases

1. Introduction

Dogs and cats have been human companions for more than 10,000 years. They have been sharing our environment and have gained a major status as "pets" in our modern, very urbanized society. Since the middle of the 20th century, they are more and more considered as "family members" within households; not to mention sometimes as substitutes for children. However, cats and dogs still can be a source of human infection by various pathogens, including viruses, bacteria, parasites, and fungi. The present manuscript analyzes and reviews the zoonotic pathogens that have recently emerged (or re-emerged) from our companion animals. This review excludes the impact of exotic and pocket pets, which deserve a distinct review.

Pet dog and cat populations have substantially increased in the developed world and it is estimated that dogs and cats are present in more than 50% of households in the USA (2012 estimated dog population: 71 million, 2012 estimated cat population: 74 million [1] and Europe (2012 estimated dog population: 75 million, 2012 estimated cat population: 90 million; with 70 million households owning a pet [2]. A similar trend is emerging in Asia in countries such as Japan, Taiwan and even China, as the Chinese population owning dogs and cats increased from 5% and 14%, respectively, in 1999 to an estimated 7% and 15% in 2004, respectively [3].

2. Viral Zoonoses

2.1. Rabies

Despite the fact that canine rabies has come under control in many parts of the developed world, it is still a major problem with pet dogs and to a lesser extent pet cats in many other parts of the world. More than 99% of human cases of rabies are still related to dog exposure [4]. An example of such an emergence or re-emergence is illustrated by the introduction of rabies in the Island of Bali, Indonesia, in 2008, leading to more than 130 human deaths [5]. Similarly, countries that have eradicated dog rabies are not exempt of accidental re-introduction by pet trade or adoption of dogs (often puppies) in rabies endemic countries and brought back home [6]. Such cases have been reported in countries such as France [7] or the USA [8]. Rabies vaccination of dogs is still the key control measure to prevent the dispersal of rabies.

2.2. Cowpox

Cowpox is an old disease that gained fame when it was shown by Jenner that it was protecting young farmers from smallpox and led to the first human vaccine. Rather uncommon now in cattle in developed countries, it has been demonstrated that in fact rodents are the natural reservoir of the virus, cows being victims of the viral infection, just like humans [9]. However, more human cases are now related to cat exposure in the United Kingdom or Western Europe. For domestic cats, more than 400 cases of cowpox infections have been described [10]. Both animals and humans reveal local exanthema on arms and legs or on the face. Although cowpox is generally regarded as a self-limiting disease, immunosuppressed patients can develop a lethal systemic disease resembling smallpox. In domestic cats, multiple skin lesions (primarily seen on head, oral cavity, neck, forelimb, or paws), conjunctivitis, or purulent ocular discharge develop upon infection. Systemic infections may occur if inner organs as the lungs (necrotizing pneumonia), co-infections or immune-deficiency are involved [10]. It is estimated that more than 50% of human cases of cowpox in the United Kingdom are related to exposure to cats [11].

2.3. Avian Influenza

Cases of influenza H5N1 have been reported in domestic cats in Europe (Austria, Germany) and several countries in Asia [12]. An outbreak was also reported in captive tigers in a Zoological garden in Thailand. These tigers had been fed with chickens that died of avian influenza H5N1 [12]. A few cases of cats infected with H1N1 in the USA [13] and Italy [14] have also been reported. An outbreak of avian influenza H3N2 was reported in pet dogs in South Korea in 2007. The epidemic of H3N8 in greyhounds in the USA is related to an equine influenza virus and has not been shown to be zoonotic. The role of cats and dogs as a source of human infection seems limited. However, cats were fully susceptible to experimental infection and infected cats were able to infect naive cats. The role of dogs seem even more limited for the dispersal of avian influenza to humans. Rather, humans may be the source of pet infection, as suggested for H1N1 infection [13].

2.4. Noroviruses, Rotaviruses

There are only anecdotal links exist between dog gastrointestinal viruses and human infections. Human norovirus (NoV) sequences were recently detected in fecal samples from pet dogs that had been in direct contact with humans with NoV gastroenteritis, suggesting that human NoVs can at least survive in the gastrointestinal tract of dogs [15]. However, canine noroviruses (CaNoV) have also been recently identified [16] and a few reports have suggested the role of dogs in the dispersal of noroviruses. CaNoV may infect humans, and small animal veterinarians are at an increased risk, as antibodies to CaNoV were found in 22.3% of 373 small animal veterinarians and 5.8% of 120 age-matched control individuals [17]. A report of infection by an animal-like strain of rotavirus (PA260/97) was diagnosed in a child with gastroenteritis in Palermo, Italy, in 1997. Sequence analysis of VP7, VP4, VP6, and NSP4 genes showed resemblance to a G3P [6] canine strain identified in Italy in 1996 [18]. Similarly, a strain similar to a rare canine strain G3P [6] was also detected from a one year old child in Brazil [19].

3. Bacterial Zoonoses

3.1. Bite-Transmitted Bacterial Infections

Pasteurella multocida, Capnocytophaga canimorsus are among the emerging or re-emerging pathogens that cause severe diseases in high-risk groups: immunocompromised individuals, elderly people, organ transplant recipients, or cancer patients [20,21]. New modes of infection have been identified in recent years either by kissing pets, giving palliative care, or sleeping with the pets [22–24]. For *C. canimorsus*, the bacterial isolates are classifiable into two main groups (I and II) with differing γ-glutamyl aminopeptidase activity [25]. Strains from human patients belonged unevenly to group I, possibility suggesting that group I can be transmitted to humans, and group II is indigenous only to the oral cavities of dogs and cats [25].

3.2. Cat Scratch Disease

Bartonella henselae has been identified only in the early 1990s as the etiological agent of cat scratch disease (CSD), causing fever and enlarged lymph nodes in humans [26]. In less than 15% of the CSD cases, complicated forms, including visceral lesions, encephalitis and endocarditis have been reported. In immunocompromised individuals, it causes bacillary angiomatosis characterized by cutaneous vasculo-proliferative lesions that can be fatal if not properly treated with antibiotics (doxycycline, gentamycine, erythromycin) for several weeks to three months [27]. Cat fleas are the main vector and transmit infection through flea feces containing infective bacteria, which can survive several days in the environment. Cats transmit the infection to humans through scratches when infective flea feces contaminate their claws. Stray cats and young cats are more likely to be bacteremic and being a source of human infection [26]. The role of dogs as source of human infection is not yet clearly understood, as dogs can be infected by a wide range of *Bartonella* species, besides *B. henselae*.

3.3. Methicillin Resistant Staphylococcus Aureus (MRSA) Infection

Staphylococcus aureus is a common human commensal organism; acquisition of genes encoding an altered penicillin-binding protein confers resistance to beta-lactam antimicrobial drugs. Methicillin-resistant *S. aureus* (MRSA) is often resistant to non-beta-lactam antimicrobial drugs as well. Originally described as an important cause of nosocomial infection, MRSA colonization and infection are now often identified in humans outside healthcare settings [28]. Dogs and cats are more likely to be colonized/infected with *Staphylococcus pseudointermedius* than *S. aureus*, but this pathogen can acquire genes encoding methicillin resistance (*i.e.*, MRSP). Diagnosis of MRSA or MRSP has implications not only for treatment of infected animals, but also for potential zoonotic transmission. There are increasing reports that suggest pet animals may play a role in household MRSA transmission [29,30].

In the United Kingdom, the genomes of 46 multilocus sequence type (ST) 22 MRSA isolates from cats and dogs were sequenced and compared to an extensive population framework of human isolates from the same lineage [31]. Phylogenomic analyses showed that all companion animal isolates were interspersed throughout the MRSA-15 (EMRSA-15) pandemic clade and clustered with human isolates from the United Kingdom, with human isolates basal to those from companion animals, suggesting a human source for isolates infecting companion animals.

A recent study evaluated the prevalence and risk factors for MRSA carriage by pets residing in households with an MRSA-infected person [32]. Ninety-nine pets (47 dogs and 52 cats) from 66 households in which an MRSA-infected patient resided, were screened using a swab protocol and isolates from pets and humans were genotyped using two techniques and compared for concordance. Eleven (11.5%) pets representing 9 (13.6%) households were MRSA-positive, but in only six of these households were the human and animal-source strains genetically concordant. Human infection by strain USA 100 was significantly associated with pet carriage (OR = 11.4 (95% CI 1.7, 76.9); $p = 0.013$). However, the source of MRSA to the pet cannot always be attributed to the human patient. Moreover, the rapid attrition of the odds of obtaining a positive culture from pets over time suggests that MRSA carriage may be fleeting. In conclusion, as stated by Bramble *et al.* [33], "Future work to more clearly elucidate the role of pet animals should be emphasized with resultant endeavors to test interventions to curb the transmission of MRSA between humans and pet animals".

3.4. Leptospirosis

Leptospirosis is a common zoonotic disease affecting dogs and humans. However, it has re-emerged in several parts of the world, associated with both climatic changes and changes in serovars implicated in canine cases. Canine leptospirosis has been described as having re-emerged in North America around the mid-1990s, with a change in the epidemiology of the infecting serovars responsible for the disease emergence [34]. In a retrospective study of 1406 leptospirosis cases in dogs from Ontario, Canada, for the period 1998 to 2006, Alton *et al.* [34] showed a distinctive seasonal pattern of leptospirosis, with more cases occurring during the summer and fall. The temporal trend analysis was consistent with an increasing proportion or re-emergence of seropositive cases of canine leptospirosis since 1998, suggesting that the putative increase in canine leptospirosis has been genuine. Similarly, the Veterinary Medical Database of hospitals showed that the prevalence of leptospirosis in dogs in the USA and Canada, after a marked decrease in the 1970s and low levels in the 1980s, began increasing in the 1990s [35]. Hospital prevalence significantly increased in dogs between 2 and 9.9 years of age ($p < 0.05$) and in male dogs ($p < 0.05$) in each decade since the 1980s. Among weight groups in the most recent decade (2000–2009), dogs weighing <15 pounds had the greatest odds of being diagnosed with leptospirosis ($p = 0.003$). One of the major issues with canine leptospirosis, is that most of the dogs with the disease had sera reacting to serogroups other than icterohaemorrhagiae and canicola, which are contained in the vaccines, as reported in southern Germany [36] or in the USA [37]. In California, infection with *L. pomona* and *L. bratislava* was recognized as a cause of leptospirosis in dogs, which resulted in development of acute renal failure with various degrees of azotemia. Thus, available vaccines in the USA or in Europe did not protect against the most common Leptospira organisms associated with clinical disease. The recent introduction of tetravalent vaccine should help reduce such a risk.

The recommended treatment for optimal clearance of the organism from renal tubules is doxycycline, 5 mg/kg p.o. q12h, for 14 days. Annual vaccination can prevent leptospirosis caused by serovars included in the vaccine and is recommended for dogs at risk of infection.

3.5. Tuberculosis (Mycobacterium bovis, M. tuberculosis and M. microti)

The re-emergence in the United Kingdom, Northern Ireland, and in New Zealand of *Mycobacterium bovis*, the causative agent of bovine tuberculosis (bTB), has led to infection of a broad range of mammalian species in addition to domestic cattle, badgers and Australian brushtail possums (*Trichosurus vulpecula*) [38,39]. Since specific tuberculosis legislation was introduced in 2006 in Great Britain, the organism has been increasingly identified in domestic species other than cattle. Diagnostic submissions for mycobacterial culture between 2004 and 2010 showed infection in several mammals, including 116 cats, and seven dogs [39]. Gunn-Moore *et al.* [40] reviewed mycobacterial submissions to AHVLA between 2005–2008 and found *M. microti* in 19% of reported cases, with *M. bovis* in 15%. In Great Britain, isolations of *M. bovis*, *M. microti*, and *M. avium* in cats appear to have discrete, almost entirely non-overlapping geographical distributions, with *M. bovis* isolations concentrated in areas where the bTB is endemic in cattle. Cats commonly presented with single or multiple cutaneous lesions (74%), which were sometimes ulcerated or discharging, located most frequently on the head (54%). Lymph nodes were usually involved (47%), typically the submandibular nodes. Systemic or pulmonary signs were rarely seen (10%–16%). Dog tuberculosis is now less frequently reported. However, transmission of *M. tuberculosis* from infected humans to dogs may still occur, as reported in a few cases in the USA and Europe [41–43].

3.6. Kennel Cough (Bordetella bronchiseptica)

Several human cases of *Bordetella bronchiseptica* infections have been reported in immunocompromised individuals, especially organ transplant recipients and cancer patients who had been exposed either to dogs or cats that can be healthy carriers of this emerging zoonotic pathogen [44]. Symptoms ranged from asymptomatic carriage to severe pneumonia [45]. Although *B. bronchiseptica* infection remains a rare clinical condition among humans, it should be considered as potentially pathogenic when found in airways of immunocompromised patients.

3.7. Gastro-Intestinal Pathogens: Salmonella and Campylobacter

Recent studies have shown that dogs fed with raw meat or pig-ear treats were more likely to shed *Salmonella* and *Campylobacter* in the environment and be a source of human contamination. Lenz *et al.* [46] reported that *Campylobacter jejuni* was isolated from 1/42 (2.6%) raw meat-fed dogs. *Salmonella enterica* was isolated from 2/40 (5%) of the raw meat feeds, 6/42 (14%) of the raw meat-fed dog feces and none of the dogs that did not receive raw meat ($p = 0.001$). Similarly, nosocomial outbreaks have been reported in veterinary clinics in North America. In 1999 and 2000, three state health departments reported four outbreaks of gastrointestinal illness due to *Salmonella enterica* serotype Typhimurium in employees, clients, and client animals from three companion animal veterinary clinics and one animal shelter [47]. More than 45 persons and companion animals became ill. Four independent investigations resulted in the testing of 19 human samples and >200 animal samples; 18 persons and 36 animals were culture-positive for *S. typhimurium*. One outbreak was due to multidrug-resistant *S. typhimurium* R-type ACKSSuT, while the other three were due to multidrug-resistant *S. typhimurium* R-type ACSSuT DT104.

3.8. Vector-Borne Zoonoses

Despite the recognition of a wide number of vector borne diseases that can infect pets, such as Lyme disease, ehrlichiosis, or tick borne encephalitis, the risk from pets is not so much from direct transmission of these pathogens to humans as from than their role as carriers of these vectors in the shared environment. For this main reason, these zoonotic pathogens are not presented in detail in this review. Two examples are the role of dogs and cats as source of plague caused by *Yersinia pestis* after sleeping with flea infested pets [22] or the presence of dogs and brown dog ticks (*Rhipicephalus sanguineus*) in playgrounds (under the houses) leading to several cases of Rocky mountain spotted fever cases in Arizona [48].

4. Parasitic and Fungal Zoonoses

4.1. Echinococcosis

The life cycle of *Echinococcus multilocularis* mainly involves foxes and their rodent prey in ecosystems generally separate from humans [49]. However, as fox and coyote populations have increasingly encroached upon suburban and urban areas, domestic dogs or cats may also become infected when they eat infected wild rodents. *E. multilocularis* is endemic in parts of Europe, much of Russia, the Central Asian republics, and Western China on the old continent and the northwestern portion of Canada, and Western Alaska in the New World. In rural regions of Central North America, the cycle involves foxes and rodents of the genera *Peromyscus* and *Microtus*. The role of foxes in the zoonotic transmission of alveolar echinococcosis appears to be important, as demonstrated by increases in the incidence of human alveolar echinococcosis following the increase in population of foxes in certain parts of Europe.

The annual incidence in humans in endemic areas of Europe has increased from a mean of 0.10 per 100,000 during 1993–2000 to a mean of 0.26 per 100,000 during 2001–2005. There is evidence of parasites spreading from endemic to previously non-endemic areas in North America and North Island, Hokkaido, Japan, due principally to the movement or relocation of foxes and in Europe due to an increase in the fox population densities [50]. The infection of humans by the larval *E. multilocularis* is often the result of association with dogs that have eaten infected rodents. However, domestic cats may also be a potential source of human infection, as shown in Europe. In Germany, a case–control study demonstrated a higher risk of alveolar echinococcosis among individuals who owned dogs that killed game, dogs that roamed outdoors unattended, individuals who were farmers, and individuals who owned cats [51]. In Austria, a study to identify the risk of pet ownership (*i.e.*, cats and dogs) for alveolar echinococcosis investigated the habits and activities of 21 confirmed patients during the period 1967–1997 which were compared with the habits and activities of 84 controls matched by sex, age, and residence [52]. Cat ownership (odds ratio (OR) = 6.47, 95% confidence interval (CI) 1.54–27.29) and hunting (OR = 7.83, 95% CI 1.16–52.77) were independent risk factors associated with alveolar hydatid disease. In France, three (3.7%) *E. multilocularis* infested cats were detected out of 81 necropsied [53]. However, the role of cats in the transmission of *E. multilocularis* may not be as significant as once believed, as studies have shown they are much less susceptible to infection with the parasite than canids [49].

4.2. Onchocercosis

Cases of canine ocular onchocercosis, caused by *Onchocerca lupi*, have been reported worldwide, particularly in the United States and Europe. Its zoonotic role has been hypothesized on the basis of the reexamination of two cases of human ocular onchocerciasis and was confirmed in the sub-conjunctival region of the human eye in a patient from Turkey [54]. In the USA, a 22-month-old girl presented with neck pain and stiffness and magnetic resonance imaging showed an extradural mass extending from C2 through the C4 level with moderate to severe compression of the cord [55]. A left unilateral C2–C4 laminectomy was performed revealing an extradural rubbery tumor; a small biopsy was obtained. Examination of stained tissue revealed the presence of a parasitic worm that was identified as a gravid

O. lupi female; the first report of zoonotic *O. lupi* in the United States. The parasite has been reported in dogs and cats in the western United States, and from people in four cases reported from Europe.

4.3. Leishmaniasis

In North America, cutaneous leishmaniasis is endemic within south-central Texas and appears to be spreading northward into the Dallas-Fort Worth metro area, affecting humans, cats, and dogs [56]. Multiple vectors and rodent reservoir hosts exist within Texas, leading to consideration of vector-borne sand fly–based transmission as the primary means of disease spread in this area. More recently, canine visceral leishmaniasis was identified as endemic in the US foxhound population, mainly transmitted through vertical and horizontal (bites) routes in this population, although *Lutzomyia* species in the United States may be involved in transmission. Further study is necessary to determine the likelihood of vector-borne transmission of both cutaneous and visceral leishmaniasis in the United States. Diagnosis is based on qPCR to detect infection and serology to indicate the onset or presence of an antibody-based immune response to *Leishmania* spp. Treatment options include allopurinol, glucantime, and newer, less toxic formulations of amphotericin B, but none of these drugs lead to lifelong sterile cure, and recrudescence of both visceral and cutaneous disease is possible, although more common after infection with *L. infantum* (visceral) or *L. brasiliensis* (cutaneous). Evidence indicates that this disease may be further emerging because of changes in the environment and closer contact between pets and sylvatic ecosystems.

4.4. Sporotrichosis

In the United States, sporotrichosis is considered to be endemic to the Mississippi and Missouri River valleys, whereas cases have been reported infrequently in California and the southwestern United States. Zoonotic transmission has been reported from a variety of domestic and wild animals, but is most commonly associated with felines [57]. A major epidemic occurred in Rio de Janeiro, Brazil in the early 2000 where 83.4% of more than 750 people affected reported contact with cats with sporotrichosis, 56% of whom reported a cat scratch or bite [57]. During that epidemic more than 1500 feline cases were diagnosed. Outdoor cats are at highest risk for contracting sporotrichosis. Like humans, cats acquire the disease via penetrating injury by foreign body or by fighting other cats. Veterinarians and cat owners are at increased risk of contracting the disease because of the high level of transmissibility from felines to humans as compared with other animal species. The high level of contagiousness of cats with sporotrichosis is thought to arise from the typically high numbers of organisms present in the lesions. Once the organism gains entry, the typical incubation period is one week to two months in humans, with most cases manifesting within the first three weeks of exposure. The clinical forms of sporotrichosis are categorized as localized (or fixed) cutaneous, lymphocutaneous, disseminated (systemic), and pulmonary. The lymphocutaneous form is the most common clinical presentation, with a primary ulcerative lesion and subcutaneous nodules extending in a linear pattern along the lymphatic channels (sporotrichoid distribution). In cats, sporotrichosis varies from subclinical infection to severe systemic disease with hematogenous dissemination of *Sporothrix schenckii* [58]. The definitive diagnosis of sporotrichosis in both humans and cats requires recovery of the organism from culture. The drug of choice to treat these patients has been oral itraconazole.

5. Conclusions

Pet ownership brings major well-being support and the risk of zoonoses is limited when good animal care and appropriate preventive measures are applied in the human environment. However, the risks are not null and some behaviors (kissing, sleeping, being licked, or sharing food or kitchen utensils) or exposure of high-risk group persons may lead to disease carried by companion animals. Better diagnostic tools have also increased our knowledge of the zoonotic or potentially zoonotic pathogens present in our direct environment. Finally, pets represent excellent sentinels to identify the pathogens that can infect humans where they live or when people travel with them.

Conflicts of Interest

The authors declare no conflict of interest.

References

1. U.S. Pet Ownership Statistics. Available online: https://www.avma.org/KB/Resources/Statistics/Pages/Market-research-statistics-US-pet-ownership.aspx#companion (accessed on 9 July 2014).
2. Facts and Figures. Statistics Underline the Importance of Pet Animals in Society. Available online: http://www.fediaf.org/facts-figures/ (accessed on 9 July 2014).
3. China: Changing Attitudes to Pet Ownership Drive Pet Food Sales. Available online: http://www.marketresearchworld.net/content/view/281/77 (accessed on accessed on 9 July 2014).
4. Fooks, A.R.; Banyard, A.C.; Horton, D.L.; Johnson, N.; McElhinney, L.M.; Jackson, A.C. Current status of rabies and prospects for elimination. *Lancet* **2014**, doi:10.1016/S0140-6736(13)62707-5.
5. Townsend, S.E.; Sumantra, I.P.; Brum, E.; Cleaveland, S.; Crafter, S.; Dewi, A.P.; Dharma, D.M.; Dushoff, J.; Girardi, J.; Gunata, I.K.; *et al.* Designing programs for eliminating canine rabies from islands: Bali, Indonesia as a case study. *PLoS Negl. Trop. Dis.* **2013**, *7*, e2372.
6. Weng, H.Y.; Wu, P.I.; Yang, P.C.; Tsai, Y.L.; Chang, C.C. A quantitative risk assessment model to evaluate effective border control measures for rabies prevention. *Vet. Res.* **2010**, *41*, 11.
7. Gautret, P.; Ribadeau-Dumas, F.; Parola, P.; Brouqui, P.; Bourhy, H. Risk for rabies importation from North Africa. *Emerg. Infect. Dis.* **2011**, *17*, 2187–2193.
8. McQuiston, J.H.; Wilson, T.; Harris, S.; Bacon, R.M.; Shapiro, S.; Trevino, I.; Sinclair, J.; Galland, G.; Marano, N. Importation of dogs into the United States: Risks from rabies and other zoonotic diseases. *Zoonoses Public Health* **2008**, *55*, 421–426.
9. Vorou, R.M.; Papavassiliou, V.G.; Pierroutsakos, I.N. Cowpox virus infection: An emerging health threat. *Curr. Opin. Infect. Dis.* **2008**, *21*, 153–156.
10. Essbauer, S.; Pfeffer, M.; Meyer, H. Zoonotic poxviruses. *Vet. Microbiol.* **2010**, *140*, 229–236.
11. Lawn, R. Risk of cowpox to small animal practitioners. *Vet. Rec.* **2010**, *166*, 631.
12. Harder, T.C.; Vahlenkamp, T.W. Influenza virus infections in dogs and cats. *Vet. Immunol. Immunopathol.* **2010**, *134*, 54–60.
13. Sponseller, B.A.; Strait, E.; Jergens, A.; Trujillo, J.; Harmon, K.; Koster, L.; Jenkins-Moore, M.; Killian, M.; Swenson, S.; Bender, H.; *et al.* Influenza A pandemic (H1N1) 2009 virus infection in domestic cat. *Emerg. Infect. Dis.* **2010**, *16*, 534–537.

14. Fiorentini, L.; Taddei, R.; Moreno, A.; Gelmetti, D.; Barbieri, I.; de Marco, M.A.; Tosi, G.; Cordioli, P.; Massi, P. Influenza A pandemic (H1N1) 2009 virus outbreak in a cat colony in Italy. *Zoonoses Public Health* **2011**, *58*, 573–581.

15. Summa, M.; von Bonsdorff, C.H.; Maunula, L. Pet dogs—A transmission route for human noroviruses? *J. Clin. Virol.* **2012**, *10*, 244–247.

16. Martella, V.; Lorusso, E.; Decaro, N.; Elia, G.; Radogna, A.; D'Abramo, M.; Desario, C.; Cavalli, A.; Corrente, M.; Camero, M.; *et al.* Detection and molecular characterization of a canine norovirus. *Emerg. Infect. Dis.* **2008**, *10*, 1306–1308.

17. Mesquita, J.R.; Costantini, V.P.; Cannon, J.L.; Lin, S.C.; Nascimento, M.S.; Vinjé, J. Presence of antibodies against genogroup VI norovirus in humans. *Virol. J.* **2013**, *10*, 176.

18. De Grazia, S.; Martella, V.; Giammanco, G.M.; Gòmara, M.I.; Ramirez, S.; Cascio, A.; Colomba, C.; Arista, S. Canine-origin G3P[3] rotavirus strain in child with acute gastroenteritis. *Emerg. Infect. Dis.* **2007**, *13*, 1091–1093.

19. Luchs, A.; Cilli, A.; Morillo, S.G.; Carmona Rde, C.; Timenetsky Mdo, C. Rare G3P[3] rotavirus strain detected in Brazil: Possible human-canine interspecies transmission. *J. Clin. Virol.* **2012**, *54*, 89–92.

20. Gaastra, W.; Lipman, L.J. *Capnocytophaga canimorsus*. *Vet. Microbiol.* **2010**, *140*, 339–346.

21. Wilson, B.A.; Ho, M. *Pasteurella multocida*: From zoonosis to cellular microbiology. *Clin. Microbiol. Rev.* **2013**, *26*, 631–655.

22. Chomel, B.B.; Sun, B. Zoonoses in the bedroom. *Emerg. Infect. Dis.* **2011**, *17*, 167–172.

23. Kawashima, S.; Matsukawa, N.; Ueki, Y.; Hattori, M.; Ojika, K. *Pasteurella multocida* meningitis caused by kissing animals: A case report and review of the literature. *J. Neurol.* **2010**, *257*, 653–654.

24. Myers, E.M.; Ward, S.L.; Myers, J.P. Life-threatening respiratory pasteurellosis associated with palliative pet care. *Clin. Infect. Dis.* **2012**, *54*, e55–e57.

25. Umeda, K.; Hatakeyama, R.; Abe, T.; Takakura, K.; Wada, T.; Ogasawara, J.; Sanada, S.; Hase, A. Distribution of *Capnocytophaga canimorsus* in dogs and cats with genetic characterization of isolates. *Vet. Microbiol.* **2014**, *171*, 153–159.

26. Chomel, B.B.; Boulouis, H.J.; Maruyama, S.; Breitschwerdt, E.B. *Bartonella* spp. in pets and effect on human health. *Emerg. Infect. Dis.* **2006**, *12*, 389–394.

27. Rolain, J.M.; Brouqui, P.; Koehler, J.E.; Maguina, C.; Dolan, M.J.; Raoult, D. Recommendations for treatment of human infections caused by *Bartonella* species. *Antimicrob. Agents Chemother.* **2004**, *48*, 1921–1933.

28. Cohn, L.A.; Middleton, J.R. A veterinary perspective on methicillin-resistant staphylococci. *J. Vet. Emerg. Crit. Care (San Antonio)* **2010**, *20*, 31–45.

29. Faires, M.C.; Tater, K.C.; Weese, J.S. An investigation of methicillin-resistant *Staphylococcus aureus* colonization in people and pets in the same household with an infected person or infected pet. *J. Am. Vet. Med. Assoc.* **2009**, *235*, 540–543.

30. Weese, J.S.; Dick, H.; Willey, B.M.; McGeer, A.; Kreiswirth, B.N.; Innis, B.; Low, D.E. Suspected transmission of methicillin-resistant *Staphylococcus aureus* between domestic pets and humans in veterinary clinics and in the household. *Vet. Microbiol.* **2006**, *115*, 148–155.

31. Harrison, E.M.; Weinert, L.A.; Holden, M.T.G.; Welch, J.J.; Wilson, K.; Morgan, F.J.E.; Harris, S.R.; Loeffler, A.; Boag, A.K.; Peacock, S.J.; *et al.* A shared population of epidemic methicillin-resistant *Staphylococcus aureus* 15 circulates in humans and companion animals. *mBio* **2014**, *5*, e00985-13.

32. Morris, D.O.; Lautenbach, E.; Zaoutis, T.; Leckerman, K.; Edelstein, P.H.; Rankin, S.C. Potential for pet animals to harbour methicillin-resistant *Staphylococcus aureus* when residing with human MRSA patients. *Zoonoses Public Health* **2012**, *59*, 286–293.

33. Bramble, M.; Morris, D.; Tolomeo, P.; Lautenbach, E. Potential role of pet animals in household transmission of methicillin-resistant *Staphylococcus aureus*: A narrative review. *Vector Borne Zoonotic Dis.* **2011**, *11*, 617–620.

34. Alton, G.D.; Berke, O.; Reid-Smith, R.; Ojkic, D.; Prescott, J.F. Increase in seroprevalence of canine leptospirosis and its risk factors, Ontario 1998–2006. *Can. J. Vet. Res.* **2009**, *73*, 167–175.

35. Lee, H.S.; Guptill, L.; Johnson, A.J.; Moore, G.E. Signalment changes in canine leptospirosis between 1970 and 2009. *J. Vet. Intern. Med.* **2014**, *28*, 294–299.

36. Geisen, V.; Stengel, C.; Brem, S.; Müller, W.; Greene, C.; Hartmann, K. Canine leptospirosis infections—Clinical signs and outcome with different suspected *Leptospira* serogroups (42 cases). *J. Small Anim. Pract.* **2007**, *48*, 324–328.

37. Adin, C.A.; Cowgill, L.D. Treatment and outcome of dogs with leptospirosis: 36 cases (1990–1998). *J. Am. Vet. Med. Assoc.* **2000**, *216*, 371–375.

38. Baker, M.G.; Lopez, L.D.; Cannon, M.C.; de Lisle, G.W.; Collins, D.M. Continuing *Mycobacterium bovis* transmission from animals to humans in New Zealand. *Epidemiol. Infect.* **2006**, *134*, 1068–1073.

39. Broughan, J.M.; Downs, S.H.; Crawshaw, T.R.; Upton, P.A.; Brewer, J.; Clifton-Hadley, R.S. *Mycobacterium bovis* infections in domesticated non-bovine mammalian species. Part 1: Review of epidemiology and laboratory submissions in Great Britain 2004–2010. *Vet. J.* **2013**, *198*, 339–345.

40. Gunn-Moore, D.A.; McFarland, S.E.; Brewer, J.I.; Crawshaw, T.R.; Clifton-Hadley, R.S.; Kovalik, M.; Shaw, D.J. Mycobacterial disease in cats in Great Britain: I. Culture results, geographical distribution and clinical presentation of 339 cases. *J. Feline Med. Surg.* **2011**, *13*, 934–944.

41. Erwin, P.C.; Bemis, D.A.; McCombs, S.B.; Sheeler, L.L.; Himelright, I.M.; Halford, S.K.; Diem, L.; Metchock, B.; Jones, T.F.; Schilling, M.G.; *et al.* *Mycobacterium tuberculosis* transmission from human to canine. *Emerg. Infect. Dis.* **2004**, *10*, 2258–2210.

42. Hackendahl, N.C.; Mawby, D.I.; Bemis, D.A.; Beazley, S.L. Putative transmission of *Mycobacterium tuberculosis* infection from a human to a dog. *J. Am. Vet. Med. Assoc.* **2004**, *225*, 1573–1577, 1548.

43. Posthaus, H.; Bodmer, T.; Alves, L.; Oevermann, A.; Schiller, I.; Rhodes, S.G.; Zimmerli, S. Accidental infection of veterinary personnel with *Mycobacterium tuberculosis* at necropsy: A case study. *Vet. Microbiol.* **2011**, *149*, 374–380.

44. Ner, Z.; Ross, L.A.; Horn, M.V.; Keens, T.G.; MacLaughlin, E.F.; Starnes, V.A.; Woo, M.S. *Bordetella bronchiseptica* infection in pediatric lung transplant recipients. *Pediatr. Transplant.* **2003**, *7*, 413–417.

45. Wernli, D.; Emonet, S.; Schrenzel, J.; Harbarth, S. Evaluation of eight cases of confirmed Bordetella bronchiseptica infection and colonization over a 15-year period. *Clin. Microbiol. Infect.* **2011**, *17*, 201–203.

46. Lenz, J.; Joffe, D.; Kauffman, M.; Zhang, Y.; LeJeune, J. Perceptions, practices, and consequences associated with food-borne pathogens and the feeding of raw meat to dogs. *Can. Vet. J.* **2009**, *50*, 637–643.

47. Wright, J.G.; Tengelsen, L.A.; Smith, K.E.; Bender, J.B.; Frank, R.K.; Grendon, J.H.; Rice, D.H.; Thiessen, A.M.; Gilbertson, C.J.; Sivapalasingam, S.; *et al.* Multidrug-resistant *Salmonella Typhimurium* in four animal facilities. *Emerg. Infect. Dis.* **2005**, *11*, 1235–1241.

48. Nicholson, W.L.; Paddock, C.D.; Demma, L.; Traeger, M.; Johnson, B.; Dickson, J.; McQuiston, J.; Swerdlow, D. Rocky Mountain spotted fever in Arizona: Documentation of heavy environmental infestations of *Rhipicephalus sanguineus* at an endemic site. *Ann. N. Y. Acad. Sci.* **2006**, *1078*, 338–341.

49. Moro, P.; Schantz, P.M. Echinococcosis: A review. *Int. J. Infect. Dis.* **2009**, *13*, 125–133.

50. Deplazes, P.; van Knapen, F.; Schweiger, A.; Overgaauw, P.A. Role of pet dogs and cats in the transmission of helminthic zoonoses in Europe, with a focus on echinococcosis and toxocarosis. *Vet. Parasitol.* **2011**, *182*, 41–53.

51. Kern, P.; Ammon, A.; Kron, M.; Sinn, G.; Sander, S.; Petersen, L.R.; Gaus, W.; Kern, P. Risk factors for alveolar echinococcosis in humans. *Emerg. Infect. Dis.* **2004**, *10*, 2088–2093.

52. Kreidl, P.; Allerberger, F.; Judmaier, G.; Auer, H.; Aspöck, H.; Hall, A.J. Domestic pets as risk factors for alveolar hydatid disease in Austria. *Am. J. Epidemiol.* **1998**, *147*, 978–981.

53. Petavy, A.F.; Tenora, F.; Deblock, S.; Sergent, V. *Echinococcus multilocularis* in domestic cats in France. A potential risk factor for alveolar hydatid disease contamination in humans. *Vet. Parasitol.* **2000**, *87*, 151–156.

54. Otranto, D.; Sakru, N.; Testini, G.; Gürlü, V.P.; Yakar, K.; Lia, R.P.; Dantas-Torres, F.; Bain, O. Case report: First evidence of human zoonotic infection by *Onchocerca lupi* (Spirurida, Onchocercidae). *Am. J. Trop. Med. Hyg.* **2011**, *84*, 55–58.

55. Eberhard, M.L.; Ostovar, G.A.; Chundu, K.; Hobohm, D.; Feiz-Erfan, I.; Mathison, B.A.; Bishop, H.S.; Cantey, P.T. Zoonotic *Onchocerca lupi* infection in a 22-month-old child in Arizona: First report in the United States and a review of the literature. *Am. J. Trop. Med. Hyg.* **2013**, *88*, 601–605.

56. Petersen, C.A. Leishmaniasis, an emerging disease found in companion animals in the United States. *Top. Companion Anim Med.* **2009**, *24*, 182–188.

57. Rees, R.K.; Swartzberg, J.E. Feline-transmitted sporotrichosis: A case study from California. *Dermatol. Online J.* **2011**, *17*, 2.

58. Schubach, A.; Barros, M.B.; Wanke, B. Epidemic sporotrichosis. *Curr. Opin. Infect. Dis.* **2008**, *21*, 129–133.

3

Public Attitudes toward Animal Research: A Review

Elisabeth H. Ormandy * and Catherine A. Schuppli

Animal Welfare Program, University of British Columbia, 2357 Main Mall, Vancouver, British Columbia, V6T 1Z4, Canada; E-Mail: schuppli@mail.ubc.ca

* Author to whom correspondence should be addressed; E-Mail: ehormandy@gmail.com.

Simple Summary: Public engagement on issues related to animal research, including exploration of public attitudes, provides a means of achieving socially acceptable scientific practice and oversight through an understanding of societal values and concerns. Numerous studies have been conducted to explore public attitudes toward animal use, and more specifically the use of animals in research. This paper reviews relevant literature using three categories of influential factors: personal and cultural characteristics, animal characteristics, and research characteristics.

Abstract: The exploration of public attitudes toward animal research is important given recent developments in animal research (e.g., increasing creation and use of genetically modified animals, and plans for progress in areas such as personalized medicine), and the shifting relationship between science and society (*i.e.*, a move toward the democratization of science). As such, public engagement on issues related to animal research, including exploration of public attitudes, provides a means of achieving socially acceptable scientific practice and oversight through an understanding of societal values and concerns. Numerous studies have been conducted to explore public attitudes toward animal use, and more specifically the use of animals in research. This paper reviews relevant literature using three categories of influential factors: personal and cultural characteristics, animal characteristics, and research characteristics. A critique is given of survey style methods used to collect data on public attitudes, and recommendations are given on how best to address current gaps in public attitudes literature.

Keywords: animals and society; animal experimentation; governance; public engagement

1. Introduction

The use of animals in research fosters a diverse range of attitudes, with some people expressing desire for complete abolition of animal research practices, while others express strong support [1–4]. However, as Knight *et al.* [5] point out, the fundamental arguments used to oppose or support animal research have shifted little over time: typically, those who oppose animal research tend to focus on animal welfare and the suffering of the animals involved, whereas those who are involved in research (e.g., scientists, researchers) tend to base their arguments on the benefits of their work and the lack of alternatives to animal models [6,7].

In previous public attitudes literature, there is often no distinction made between different types of animal use and there appears to be an underlying assumption that people's attitudes are uni-dimensional [8]. Typically, public attitudes studies involve the use of survey style methods; however, some studies do not disclose all the methodological details of the survey [9], and in some cases the questions that make up these surveys are worded in biased ways, thus compromising the value of the results.

The case is often made that the public does not have enough background knowledge to be involved in discussions or engagement exercises about animal research—the so-called deficit or 'Enlightenment' model [10]. Whilst having some support in studies that show a relationship between familiarity with science and support for animal research, e.g., [11–15], the deficit model has nevertheless been widely criticized. Indeed, one study has shown that as knowledge increases members of the public may become less supportive, particularly if the topic under discussion is considered morally contentious, e.g., [16]. Other studies have echoed this and found that in some cases familiarity with animal research was associated with lower levels of support, e.g., [12,14,17,18]. Furthermore, some authors propose that science and society cannot feasibly be separated, and have called for the democratization of scientific practice [10,19,20]. Since there are shifts toward the democratization of science [21], it becomes increasingly important to understand public attitudes toward scientific practices that invoke polarized opinion or might be considered morally contentious, such as animal research, and to develop novel mechanisms for public engagement on such issues.

The term 'attitude' has been used to refer to "the evaluation of an object, concept, or behaviour along a dimension of favour or disfavour, good or bad, like or dislike" [22] (p. 3). Attitudes are distinct from, but related to, people's beliefs and values. It is postulated in the expectancy-value model [23,24] that attitudes are formed through a person's accessible beliefs about an object, where a belief is defined as "the subjective probability that the object has a certain attribute"[22]. Azjen and Fishbein [22] (p. 4) give an illustrative example: "a person may believe that exercise (the attitude object) reduces the risk of heart disease (the attribute)." An important implication of the expectancy-value model is that attitudes towards an object are formed automatically and inevitably as we acquire new (and pertinent) information about an object's attributes, and as the subjective values of these attributes become linked to the object [24]. Therefore, assessing people's attitudes towards animals and animal research can tell us more about whether different types of animal research are normatively considered 'good' or 'bad' at both a personal and societal level.

There are several factors that previous literature has shown to influence people's attitudes towards animals, and animal-based research specifically (as identified by Knight and Barnett [8]): personal and cultural characteristics, animal characteristics, and research characteristics. By exploring these influential factors in detail the following review provides an update on the survey-based public attitudes literature that was reviewed a decade ago by Hagelin *et al.* [4]. The authors then go on to discuss shortcomings associated with survey style methods in more depth. Finally, in light of this critique, the paper makes recommendations on how gaps in this growing literature can be addressed to move toward more sound models of public engagement.

2. Personal and Cultural Characteristics

In order to understand different attitudes toward the human use of animals, and their use in research specifically, many studies have focused on personal characteristics: that is, things about a person that may influence their decision on whether to support or oppose the use of animals in research. The personal characteristics discussed below include: age, sex, rural *versus* urban background, experience of animals/pet ownership, and religion. Also discussed are factors based more on a person's beliefs and potentially shaped by personal characteristics: vegetarianism, and belief in animal mind.

2.1. Age

It has generally been reported that moral acceptance of the use of animals in research is positively correlated with age [4]. In their 1981 study [25], Kellert and Berry suggest that younger people are more opposed to animal use than older people. The authors go on to describe how older males presented a more instrumental view toward animals, suggesting that older people tend to emphasize the practical value of animals. Other studies have echoed this finding [17,26–28]. However, some studies have found, conversely, that younger participants are more supportive of animal-based research that older participants, e.g., [11]. The effect of age on attitudes toward animals may be a cohort effect, where people with a shared history are more likely to share beliefs and attitudes [29], or may be also be related to attitudinal change with age [30].

2.2. Sex

Sex identity has been consistently found to relate to attitudes toward the treatment of research animals (and animals in general), with virtually all studies reporting that women are more likely to object to animal use [12,25,26,31,32]. A lower proportion of women accept the use of animals in research compared to men [27,33–37] and most studies of the animal protection movement have found that women activists outnumber men by a ratio of two or three to one [38–40]. The effects of sex identity on attitudes toward the use of animals in research are consistent across many studies, with differences between males and females extending to at least 15 different countries [14]. Pifer [15] reported that, among a range of predictors, sex identity was the strongest correlate of opposition to animal research.

It might be that females are less supportive of animal use because they are more likely to attribute mental states to animals, and more likely to have a sympathetic reaction if they believe that animal use will cause some kind of pain or distress to animals [18]. Indeed, males have been shown to present lower levels of belief in the mental abilities of animals compared to females [41] (see later paragraph for a discussion of belief in animal mind). In addition Kellert [42] reported that men exhibited more "dominionistic" attitudes toward the environment, while women exhibited more "moralistic" attitudes, a difference that might also explain sex difference in attitudes toward animal use.

Rather than characterizing people strictly by biologically determined sex, others have examined sex role orientation (SRO) in relation to attitudes toward the use of animals in research [43,44]. Herzog *et al.* [43] suggest that differences in attitudes are associated with feminine *versus* masculine SRO, with people who identify as more feminine being generally less supportive. However, Peek *et al.* [44] speculate that sex differences differ not as a result of SRO, but because of the structural location of females in society (*i.e.*, females may perceive themselves and animals to have similar positions in society; [45]). Similarly, women's social positions may also lead to greater concern for animals. For example, Kendall *et al.* [29] argue that women are typically primary family caretakers (and so are more likely to take on nurturing roles), and may be more likely to engage in household tasks that put them in more direct contact with animals.

2.3. Rural versus Urban Background

Some studies have shown that people with a rural background have a greater acceptance of animal use than urban people, and greater support for animal experimentation [14,46,47]. This finding suggests that rural and urban places provide distinct opportunities for contact and relationships with animals, as well as diverse cultural experiences that shape and strengthen people's attitudes about animals [29]. Animal use often differs in urban and rural regions [39]. The instrumental relationships with animals that are associated with rural settings might shape an individual's attitudes toward animals in different contexts, including animal research. A cross-cultural study of people's attitudes toward the use of animals in research [14] found that there was a link between a nation's level of industrialization and urbanization and attitudes toward animal research. For instance, the two least industrialized countries within the European Community had the highest level of support for animal research. Crettaz von Roten [13] also found differences in acceptance of animal research between European countries, with industrialized countries (*i.e.*, countries where labor is more physical in nature) displaying higher levels of approval of animal research than post-industrial countries (*i.e.*, countries where labor is more mental in nature). Pifer *et al.* [14] suggest that countries that have closer relationship with the land have more pragmatic and utilitarian attitudes about animals, such that the use of animals by humans in not seen as contentious. In developed countries urban people may never come into contact with the animals they eat; instead, animals are more likely to be companions and part of the family [39]. Perhaps for this reason, urban residence has been found to be related to greater concern for animal well-being [31,46,48].

2.4. Experience with Animals

Attitudes toward the human use of animals can also be shaped by a person's previous or existing experience of animals [8,35]; for example, Driscoll [26] found that pet owners rated animal-based research as less acceptable than did non-pet owners. This finding is also echoed in other studies that showed that pet owners form an attachment with their animals, and that this strengthens a general positive attitude toward other animals [49–52]. According to 'contact theory', e.g., [53], contact with members of an 'outgroup' (e.g., non-human animals) can lead to a mutual understanding and decreased prejudice toward that group. Contact may also foster emotional attachment and empathy toward animals [54–57]. This may explain why positive experiences of animals promote affection and positive attitudes toward animals in general, which is in conflict with utility or instrumental uses of animals, such as research animals [58]. Thus pet ownership, or other positive experiences of animals may increase people's opposition to animal research. Conversely, a negative encounter with an animal may equally shape people's views, making them more supportive of animal use [59]. In addition, the type of contact that an individual has with animals may also influence their attitudes towards animals: as previously mentioned, contact with animals through circumstances such as farming may promote a more instrumental view towards animals, rather than one based on companionship.

2.5. Religion

Religion can influence how people view and relate to animals. For example, Christianity has been shown to be positively associated with support for the use of animals in research [60]. Driscoll [26] found differing views across different Christian denominations: persons reporting no religious affiliation or an affiliation with the Catholic church rated various examples of animal-based research as less acceptable than did persons reporting a traditional Protestant affiliation. There are, of course, also specific animal species that are either revered (e.g., cows in Hinduism) or avoided (e.g., pigs in Judaism) in different religious traditions. This may in turn affect people's willingness to support or oppose the use of certain species for research purposes.

2.6. Personality

An individual's personality type, and the way in which people morally evaluate situations can influence their willingness to support animal research. Previous literature has classified people into four ethical perspectives: absolutists (high idealism, low relativism), situationists (high idealism, high relativism), exceptionists (low idealism, low relativism), and subjectivists (low idealism, high relativism) [61]. Working with this framework, Galvin and Herzog [62] have illustrated that absolutism (high idealism) is high amongst animal activists, as opposed to subjectivism (low idealism), which was low. In a separate study, Galvin and Herzog [63] also showed that idealism was high amongst participants who rejected hypothetical animal research proposals. These findings were further echoed in a study by Wuensch and Poteat [64] in which different types of animal research proposals were approved by participants who were significantly less idealistic and significantly more relativistic. Overall, evidence to date suggests that support for animal research is negatively associated with personality types that tend towards idealism, and positively associated with relativism.

2.7. Vegetarianism and Animal or Environmental Advocacy

Vegetarianism has been associated with lower acceptance of the use of animals in research compared to non-vegetarianism [11,17,50]. Demand for particular types of food is influenced primarily by social and psychological factors such as beliefs, attitudes, norms, and values [46], and vegetarianism is related to value orientations such as an increase in altruistic values and a decrease in traditional (*i.e.*, instrumental) values [65]. Moreover, vegetarianism is likely to relate to a wider ideological perspective in terms of the 'world view' or 'ethical ideology' held by people [27,66,67]. So, rather than being a predictor of attitudes toward animals *per se*, vegetarianism is an action or behaviour that results from a particular attitude toward animals. This attitude may be generalized into a broader concern with animal rights, protection or welfare, due to underlying beliefs, meaning that vegetarian individuals are more likely to oppose the use of animals in research.

In a similar vein, an interest in environmental issues (which may also be linked to vegetarianism) is negatively related to support for animal research [12]. Studies have shown that people who are politically left-wing-oriented are less supportive of animal experimentation. This finding may also be explained by differences in people's worldviews or ethical ideologies [9,66,68], because attitudes toward animals are closely related to attitudes toward other political and social matters [27].

2.8. Belief in Animal Mind

"Belief in animal mind" (BAM) is the term used to describe people's belief in the mental abilities of animals. Does one believe that animals are self-aware, capable of solving problems, or experiencing emotions such as fear, sadness, happiness and pleasure? [18,41]. BAM is a relatively consistent predictor of attitudes toward the human use of animals [18,41,46,69], and in one small qualitative study BAM appeared to explain more of the variation in people's attitudes than personal characteristics, such as sex [8]. BAM negatively correlates with support for animal use and positively correlates with concern for animal welfare and humane behaviour toward animals [8,12], and empathy toward other humans and animals [46]. If one believes that certain species are likely to experience internal thoughts and feelings, then subjecting them to discomfort as part of animal-based research may seem unacceptable. This line of reasoning would suggest that people should be less accepting of research using species rated highly in BAM, particularly non-human primates. However, a study by Knight *et al.* [5] showed that more support was expressed for the use of monkeys in medical research compared to other animals, such as dogs, cats, rabbits, guinea pigs, rats and mice. In this study it was scientists (rather than lay persons or animal welfarists) who indicated strong support for the use of monkeys in research. Knight *et al.* [5] show that, despite attributing 'animal mind' to monkeys, scientists' perception was that monkeys are more appropriate animal models for medical research practice. This finding shows that, in some cases, BAM may be trumped by other factors (such as perceived benefit or necessity of research).

3. Animal Characteristics

While most studies have focused on personal and cultural characteristics to explain variation in attitudes, factors relating to animal characteristics also influence people's view on this subject. The animal characteristics discussed below include species, sentience, neoteny/appeal and genetic modification.

3.1. Species, Sentience and Appeal

People hold different attitudes toward animal use depending on the species involved [26,41,70]. People tend to rate animals classed as pets (e.g., dogs and cats) or non-human primates as having higher mental abilities compared to other species such as fish or mice [41,71]. People are more supportive of using smaller-brained animals such as mice and rats [71], and less supportive of using animals classed as pets [26], and animals believed to have 'higher' mental abilities enabling them to use tools, solve problems, and be self aware [8,41]. Therefore, the same person may support the use of mice and rats for dissection purposes, but not support the use of chimpanzees, cats or dogs for the same purpose. In a recent study involving interviews with members of animal care committees (responsible for the ethical review of research proposals involving the use of live animals) Schuppli [69] reported that committee members were less comfortable with research using non-human primates and companion animals. Different views regarding species may be due to a belief in the mentality of different species, or their human-like qualities in terms of human experience [69,72] as well as other factors such as personal affection for particular kinds of animals, or individual animals [73], the special consideration given to certain species based on the relationship we typically have with those animals [35,74], where the species falls on the phylogenetic scale [75], or their 'cuteness' or attractiveness [4,8,41]. From literature on public attitudes toward species conservation, it has also been shown that animals that retain a neonatal appearance (neoteny) are more likely to be supported in conservation efforts [76,77].

However, it is not always the case that animal research using species that are lower on the phylogentic scale is more acceptable. In a study asking participants about their willingness to support the use of animals to create models of skin cancer, there was no species effect of switching from zebrafish to mice (despite predictions that support would drop when fish were replaced with mammals [78]). Attitudes toward the use of different species in research may also change as we learn more about animal behaviour and welfare; for example, recent research suggests that fish (that are often considered an acceptable replacement for mammals in research [79–81]) have the capacity to feel pain [82,83].

3.2. Genetic Modification

Public views toward the genetic modification of animals tend to be complex, but predominantly negative [84]. Genetic modification of animals presents new challenges in terms of maintaining public acceptance of animal-based research. Some members of the public express grave concern for the 'unnaturalness' of genetic modification and its potential to lead to unknown consequences [17,68,85]. Indeed, people's perception of what is "natural" has been shown to decrease with the alteration of genetic material through genetic engineering [86]. In his 2001 study, Macnaghten [85] found considerable concern about genetic modification and the uses to which genetically modified (GM) animals might be put. Participants in his focus-group study showed a "reaction against the proposed technology as intrinsically a violation of nature and transgressive of so-called natural parameters" [85] (p. 25)—what might be called the "yuk response" [87]. Such findings are echoed in other studies, e.g., [26,88]. Another primary concern that has emerged is that genetic modification might lead to unexpected (and potentially bad) consequences; indeed, one aspect of the unease about GM animals is a fear that nature might 'bite back' [84,89]. In addition to these main arguments in opposition to GM, a more recent study by Macnaghten [89] shows an emerging concern from the public about the increase in the numbers of animals used in research due to the currently inefficient and unpredictable nature of the genetic modification process. This sentiment also emerges in studies by Schuppli et al. [74] and

Ormandy *et al.* [90] who argue that the creation and use of GM animals challenges the Three Rs principles (replacement, reduction, refinement), particularly reduction.

4. Research Characteristics

The characteristics of the research that an animal will be involved in can also influence people's decisions about whether to support or oppose the research. The research characteristics discussed below are: the purpose of the research, the level of invasiveness (or harm) that the animal will experience, and availability of non-animal alternatives.

4.1. Type of Research

It is common that medical experiments involving animals are more positively regarded than experiments for cosmetics testing. For example, Aldhous *et al.* [91] found that whether or not mice were subjected to pain, illness, or surgeries, people were more likely to disapprove if the experiment was designed to test the safety of a cosmetics ingredient than if it tested the safety and effectiveness of a drug or vaccine, and this result was echoed in numerous other studies [8,14,26,64,69]. Conversely, Schuppli and Weary [11] found that participants in an online public engagement study were more supportive of the use of pigs in environmental research (to reduce agricultural pollution) than for biomedical research (to decrease rejection rates in organ transplantation). However, the purpose of the research may be trumped by other influential factors. For example, non-animal alternatives to the biomedical research scenario used in the study by Schuppli and Weary [11] (e.g., increasing human organ donations) may be seen as a more viable option. It would appear that people's attitudes toward experiments involving animals are likely to change depending on the beneficiary, purpose or necessity of the research. As noted by Henry and Pulcino [92] "the literature suggests that animal research that is viewed as providing tangible, meaningful benefits to humans is considered more acceptable than animal research that is viewed and less beneficial or necessary."

4.2. Availability of Alternatives

The perceived necessity of animal research ties into the availability of non-animal alternatives, with research that is deemed unnecessary being less favoured. For example, Stanistreet and Spofforth [93] found that participants were less supportive of the use of animals in research that was viewed as "non-necessary" than research that was viewed as "necessary." It seems that the availability of non-animal alternatives, or a belief that alternatives exist, may be particularly influential on people's attitudes toward the use of animals in research, e.g., [4]. Two studies in particular illustrate that when non-animal alternatives are available, there is higher level of opposition. Research by Knight *et al.* [18] showed that animal use was most likely to be supported when participants perceived there to be no other choice than using animals. However, Knight *et al.* [18] also found that their participants (nine men, eight women) could seldom think of alternatives to using animals in research and in teaching, and so they believed that there was little choice other than using animals. In a follow up study, Knight *et al.* [5] showed that different attitudes toward animal experimentation between scientists and animal welfarists could, in part, be explained by differing beliefs in the availability of non-animal alternatives.

4.3. Level of Harm

Invasiveness, or level of harm that the animals experience during a given experiment has also been shown to influence people's support of animal-based research [33,37]. Richmond *et al.* [94] found that the most common objection to animal experimentation is related to whether animals experience pain and suffering. In fact, a review by Hagelin *et al.* [4] illustrated that survey respondents are less likely to support animal research if the words "pain" or "death" are used. In a more recent study [92] results indicated that participants were more opposed to biomedical research that resulted in harm to animals.

In addition, Bateson [95] has made the argument that animal suffering (level of harm) should be weighed against the importance of the research, and the likelihood of benefit when making decisions about whether animal research should proceed. As described in the subsections above, these factors (especially the importance of the research) are also important to members of the public.

5. Other Variables

There are other variables that may affect people's attitudes towards animals, or animal research, that do not fit neatly into the three categories above. In particular, the effect of social media, and the living conditions of animals in laboratories have been shown to have an effect on people's attitudes.

5.1. Effect of Social Media

The use of social media by animal rights organizations has been successful in raising public awareness of certain issues related to animal research [96]—this is further illustrated by the large memberships of social media groups with an animal rights or welfare focus (e.g., PETA currently have over 2 million Facebook group members). To the author's knowledge no academic literature to date has explicitly tested the effects of social media on people's willingness to support animal research. However, one study by Kruse *et al.* [97] documented how pro-research efforts get more positive attention in social media. The authors of this study go on to argue that members of the public are the most easily influenced by social media because they are not well-informed about animal research. A different study [98] documented how public attitudes towards California's cougars were shifted and reflected over a decade (1985–1995) through print media.

5.2. Living Conditions of Laboratory Animals

In several different online engagement studies, participants were more willing to support animal research provided that their concerns about animal welfare (including the day-to-day care and handling of animals) were addressed [17,78,88]. These findings indicate that the living conditions of animals kept for research purposes can affect people's attitudes towards animal research, and if animals are well-housed and cared for, people's support for animal research will perhaps increase.

6. Critique of Existing Methods of Public Attitudes Assessment

There is a growing body of literature related to public attitudes toward animal use in general, and animal research more specifically. However there are potential shortcomings that should be addressed for future studies. Three primary shortcomings are discussed below: use of college students as participant samples, use of general questions about 'animal use' rather than specific questions about different types of animal use (or even different types of animal research), and use of Likert scales or rating scales that do not allow for more qualitative reasoning.

While numerous previous studies have engaged with a broader public membership when assessing attitudes towards animals and animal research, e.g., [13,26,35], many others have used undergraduate students (usually majoring in psychology) for their sample populations, e.g., [31,62,64,99]. In fact, Herzog and Dorr [100] examined 15 issues of Society and Animals published between 1993 and 1998 and found that, "the data in 11 of these articles were obtained using undergraduates. Of these, one article did not specify the source of the students, one used education students as subjects and the other nine were based in students taking psychology classes" [100] (p. 2). Notably, using a large national sample, Kellert [101] and Kellert and Berry [25] reported that both education and age were related to knowledge and attitudes toward animals. This suggests that college students, being both young and educated, are likely to be more concerned about animals than the general public. Given that the regulation of animals in research was developed, in part, in response to public concerns, it is pertinent that new ways of assessing attitudes toward the use of animals in research are developed that reflect a diversity of views, rather than limiting the breadth of studies by relying on convenience sampling of students. As further pointed out by Herzog and Dorr, "undergraduate psychology majors are a narrow source of information on human/animal relationships" [100] (p. 2). This is echoed in a recent article in the Economist [102], which highlights the challenges to using undergraduate students as a source of information and explores the benefits of crowd sourcing (e.g., the use of Amazon's Mechanical Turk platform to recruit survey participants). The primary benefit to crowd sourcing is the diversity of participants: there is less reliance on information provided by participants from western, educated, industrialized, rich and democratic subsets of the world population.

A second shortcoming is that most studies have asked rather general questions about animal use. Kellert and Berry [25], Driscoll [26] and Knight et al. [18] have identified this problem, showing that people have strong likes and dislikes for different kinds of animals, and multidimensional views regarding different types of animal use. To ask someone to agree or disagree with a statement such as "it is alright to do research on animals" is ambiguous. It may be that only people with more extreme views will disagree with this statement because it does not specify what kind of research, or perhaps more importantly, what kind of animals are involved.

Research animal use is changing, particularly as a result of increasing use of technologies such as genetic modification [90] and ethyl-N-nitrosourea (ENU) mutagenesis (a commonly used method of chemically inducing mutations, particularly in mice [103] and zebrafish [104]) to create animal models of disease. So far, research exploring public attitudes to genetic modification of animals has mainly focused on farm animals, rather than laboratory animals that are used in much greater numbers. Only one study to date has explored people's views toward ENU mutagenesis [78]. In addition, new developments in areas of personalized medicine, particularly oncology, may pose new challenges. For example, a patient with a tumour might be able to have tumour samples taken and implanted into animal hosts (e.g., mice) so that a range of treatments can be tested, and a better targeted therapeutic treatment for the patient developed [105]. Such procedures will likely increase animal numbers and may also require alterations to the current process of animal protocol review and approval, as well as perhaps introducing a more personal, direct involvement in the public's role in animal use.

A third shortcoming is that many of the studies cited above were performed using methods that asked participants to respond on a scale (e.g., Likert scale, rating or preference scale), or asked questions requiring a simple "Yes" or "No" response, without any insight into the reasoning that may have led to these responses. Participants are constrained in their choice of answers by the options provided by the researcher (which may lead to researcher bias) [106] and are unable to provide any qualification to explain their response. The exploration of people's reasons for their "Yes"/"No" or Likert scale responses is important. The shortcomings of restricted response options can be addressed if questions are designed with sufficient understanding of the topic: being able to ask meaningful questions that allow people to demonstrate their reasoning. Often such in-depth understanding is developed from initial qualitative research, where the quantitative research is used to confirm the findings. When restricted response options do not allow for consideration of what people's concerns are (e.g., why they might be opposed to certain types of research), it is difficult for policy makers to understand the nuance in attitudes in order to make progress in addressing societal concerns.

Aside from academic research, regular national opinion polls often ask questions about people's level of support for animal research. These polls can be valuable in tracking attitudes over time, and they invite broader perspectives from a wider and more representative sample population; however the polls remain subject to the prior criticism of using fixed response options for participants to choose from. As further pointed out by Hobson-West [107] care should be taken when referring to others' interpretation of national opinion polls, since the same posed can be used as evidence by both sides of the polarized debate about animal research.

7. Addressing the Gaps through Better Public Engagement

Pytlik Zillig and Tomkins [108] argue that public engagement is a valuable means to provide societal perspectives concerning the political, legal, ethical, and other impacts of scientific and technological research. Changes in societal attitudes often result in a push to improve animal-related regulation and public policy [109]. However, current mechanisms for including public opinion in animal research policy may be lacking. One recent article highlights the secrecy surrounding animal research [110] while another [111] draws attention to some of the problems that might be encountered if decisions about animal research are not opened up to a wider community. The case study by Lyons [111] warns against the formation of policy communities with exclusive membership that "tend(s) to produce outcomes that consistently favour network members at the expense of excluded groups" [111] (p.357). In the article, Lyons describes a specific area of research (xenotransplantation between pigs and primates) in which, to the detriment of the animals involved, decisions were made without input from experts and stakeholders outside the policy community, and without wider public engagement. Such activities go against the increasing democratization of science and science policy [10,19,21], and highlight the need for wider public engagement, especially for research that is considered to be contentious. Therefore, it is important for governing bodies to assess public opinion about animal-based research, and to engage a variety of different stakeholders, including the public, when developing animal policy.

One approach to improving public engagement on animal research issues is to conduct further empirical studies that explore public attitudes toward animal research in ways that correct for some of the criticisms outlined in this paper. For example, studies that: (1) avoid reliance on convenience sampling of students, and ensure that participants reflect a diversity of views; (2) use a well-planned experimental framework that allows exploration of not only where people draw the line in terms of what they are willing to accept, but also why; and (3) focus on gaining a better understanding of public attitudes toward specific (rather than general) aspects of animal research; for example, attitudes toward emerging technologies (like genetic modification or other genetic alteration techniques) and the most commonly used species in research (zebrafish and mice), as well as the regulatory systems that oversee animal research.

8. Summary

Various factors influence people's views toward the use of animals in research, and these can be categorized into: (1) personal and cultural characteristics; (2) animal characteristics; and (3) research characteristics. Understanding public attitudes toward the use of animals in research will facilitate the growing trend toward more openness and democratization of scientific research, and ensure that scientific practice (including animal research) remains in step with societal values. In turn, evaluating societal values and addressing societal concerns is important, as the public is often claimed to be the key beneficiary of the resulting therapeutic products that are developed and tested.

Acknowledgments

The authors are grateful to Daniel Weary for comments on draft versions of this manuscript.

Author Contributions

E. Ormandy is responsible for the generating of ideas and writing of the manuscript. C. Schuppli is responsible for helping generate ideas, for providing some of the literature cited and reviewing the manuscript.

Conflicts of Interest

The authors declare no conflict of interest.

References and Notes

1. MRC. *Views on Animal Experimentation*; MRC: London, UK, 2010. Available online: http://www.ipsos-mori.com/DownloadPublication/1343_sri-views-on-animal-experimentation-2010.pdf (accessed on 15 September 2011).
2. Gallup Poll. *Four Moral Issues Sharply Divide Americans*. 2010. Available online: http://www.gallup.com/poll/137357/Four-Moral-Issues-Sharply-Divide-Americans.aspx (accessed on 15 September 2011).
3. Eurobarometer 73.1. *Science and Technology Report*; European Union. 2010. Available online: http://ec.europa.eu/public_opinion/archives/ebs/ebs_340_en.pdf (accessed on 30 September 2011).

4. Hagelin, J.; Carlsson, H.-E.; Hau, J. An overview of surveys on how people view animal experimentation: Some factors that may influence the outcome. *Public Underst. Sci.* **2003**, *12*, 67–81.

5. Knight, S.; Vrij, A.; Bard, K.; Brandon, D. Science *versus* human welfare? Understanding attitudes towards animal use. *J. Soc. Issues* **2009**, *65*, 463–483.

6. Baldwin, E. The case for animal research in psychology. *J. Soc. Issues* **1993**, *49*, 121–131.

7. Paul, E.S. Us and them: Scientists' and animal rights campaigners' views of the animal experimentation debate. *Soc. Anim.* **1995**, *3*, 1–21.

8. Knight, S.; Barnett, L. Justifying attitudes towards animal use: A qualitative study of people's views and beliefs. *Anthrozoös* **2008**, *21*, 31–42.

9. Herzog, H.A.; Rowan, A.N.; Kossow, D. Social attitudes and animals. In *The State of the Animals*; Salem, D.J., Rowan, A.N., Eds.; Humane Society Press: Washington, DC, USA, 2001; pp. 55–69.

10. Elam, M.; Bertilsson, M. Consuming, engaging and confronting science: The emerging dimensions of scientific citizenship. *Eur. J. Soc. Theory* **2003**, *6*, 233–251.

11. Schuppli, C.A.; Weary, D.M. Attitudes towards the use of genetically modified animals in research. *Public Underst. Sci.* **2010**, *19*, 686–697.

12. Broida, J.; Tingley, L.; Kimball, R.; Miele, J. Personality differences between pro- and anti-vivisectionists. *Soc. Anim.* **1993**, *1*, 129–144.

13. Crettaz von Roten, F. Public perceptions of animal experimentation across Europe. *Public Underst. Sci.* **2013**, *22*, 691–703.

14. Pifer, L.; Shimizu, K.; Pifer, R. Public attitudes toward public research: Some international comparisons. *Soc. Anim.* **1994**, *2*, 95–113.

15. Pifer, L. Exploring the gender gap in young adults' attitudes about animal research. *Soc. Anim.* **1996**, *4*, 37–52.

16. Evans, G.; Durant, J. The relationship between knowledge and attitudes in the public understanding of science in Britain. *Public Underst. Sci.* **1995**, *4*, 57–74.

17. Ormandy, E.H.; Schuppli, C.A.; Weary, D.M. Public attitudes toward the use of animals in research: Effects of invasiveness, genetic modification and regulation. *Anthrozoös* **2013**, *26*, 165–184.

18. Knight, S.; Nunkoosing, K.; Vrig A.; Cherryman, J. Using grounded theory to examine people's attitudes towards how animals are used. *Soc. Anim.* **2003**, *11*, 179–198.

19. Irwin, A. Constructing the scientific citizen: Science and democracy in the biosciences. *Public Underst. Sci.* **2001**, *10*, 1–18.

20. Jasanoff, S. *States of Knowledge: Co-Construction of Science and Social Order*; Routledge: New York, NY, USA and London, UK, 2006.

21. Schiele, B. On and about the deficit model in an age of free flow. In *Communicating Science in Social Contexts: New Models, New Practices*; Cheng, D., Claessens, M., Gascoigne, N.R.J., Metcalfe, J., Schiele, B., Shi, S., Eds.; Springer: Berlin, Germany, 2008; pp. 93–118.

22. Ajzen, I.; Fishbein, M. Attitudes and the attitude-behavior relation: Reasoned and automatic processes. *Eur. Rev. Soc. Psychol.* **2000**, *11*, 1–33.

23. Fishbein, M. An investigation of the relationship between beliefs about an object and the attitude toward that object. *Hum. Relat.* **1963**, *16*, 233–240.

24. Fishbein, M. Attitude and the prediction of behaviour. In *Readings in Attitude Theory and Measurement*; Fishbein, M., Ed.; Wiley: New York, NY, USA, 1967; pp. 477–492.

25. Kellert, S.R.; Berry, J.K. *Knowledge, Affection and Basic Attitudes toward Animals in American Society*; PB-81-173106; National Technical Information Services: Springfield, VA, USA, 1981.

26. Driscoll, J.W. Attitudes towards animal use. *Anthrozoös* **1992**, *5*, 32–39.

27. Furnham, A.; Pinder, A. Young people's attitudes to experimentation on animals. *The Psychologist* **1990**, *October*, 444–448.

28. Medical Research Council. *Animals in Medicine and Science*; Medical Research Council: London, UK, 1999.

29. Kendall, H.A.; Lobao, L.M.; Sharp, J. Public concern with animal well-being: Place, social structural location, and individual experience. *Rural Sociol.* **2006**, *71*, 399–428.

30. Kellert, S.R. *The Value of Life: Biological Diversity and Human Society*; Island Press: Washington, DC, USA, 1996.

31. Gallup, G.G; Beckstead, J.W. Attitudes towards animal research. *Am. Psychol.* **1988**, *43*, 474–476.

32. Matthews, S.; Herzog, H.A. Personality and attitudes toward the treatment of animals. *Soc. Anim.* **1997**, *5*, 169–175.

33. Rajecki, D.W.; Rasmussen, J.L.; Craft, H.D. Labels and the treatment of animals: Archival and experimental cases. *Soc. Anim.* **1993**, *1*, 45–60.

34. Plous, S. Attitudes towards the use of animals in psychological research and education: Results from a national survey of psychology majors. *Psychol. Sci.* **1996**, *7*, 352–358.

35. Wells, D. L; Hepper, P.G. Pet ownership and adults' views on animal use. *Soc. Anim.* **1997**, *5*, 45–63.

36. Navaro, J.; Maldonado, E.; Pedraza, C.; Cavas, M. Attitudes among animal research among psychology students in Spain. *Psychol. Rep.* **2001**, *89*, 227–236.

37. Swami, V.; Furnham, A.; Christopher, A. Free the animals? Investigating attitudes toward animal testing in Britain and the United States. *Scand. J. Psychol.* **2008**, *49*, 269–276.

38. Herzog, H.A. The movement is my life: The psychology of animal rights activism. *J. Soc. Issues* **1993**, *49*, 103–119.

39. Jasper, J.; Nelkin, D. *The Animal Rights Crusade*; The Free Press: New York, NY, USA, 1992.

40. Plous, S. An attitude survey of animal rights activists. *Psychol. Sci.* **1992**, *2*, 194–196.

41. Herzog, H.A.; Galvin, S. Common sense and the mental lives of animals: An empirical approach. In *Anthropomorphism, Anecdotes and Animals*; Mitchell, R.W., Ed.; State University of New York Press: Albany, NY, USA, 1997.

42. Kellert, S.R. American attitudes towards and knowledge of animals: An update. *Int. J. Study Anim. Probl.* **1980**, *1*, 87–119.

43. Herzog, H.A.; Betchart, N.S.; Pittman, R.B. Gender, sex role orientation and attitudes towards animals. *Anthrozoös* **1991**, *4*, 184–191.

44. Peek, C.W.; Dunham, C.C.; Dietz, B.E. Gender, relational role orientation, and affinity for animal rights. *Sex Roles* **1997**, *37*, 905–920.

45. Adams, C.J. Bringing peace home: A feminist philosophical perspective on the abuse of women, children and pet animals. *Hypatia* **1994**, *9*, 63–84.

46. Hills, A.M. Empathy and belief in the mental experience of animals. Reviews and research reports. *Anthrozoös* **1995**, *8*, 132–142.

47. Kalof, L.; Dietz, T.; Stern, P.C.; Guagnano, G.A. Social psychological and structural influences on vegetarian beliefs. *Rural Sociol.* **1999**, *64*, 500–511.

48. Ohlendorf, G.W.; Jenkins, Q.A.L.; Tomazic, T.J. Who cares about farm animal welfare? In *The Social Risks of Agriculture: Americans Speak out on Food, Farming, and the Environment*; Wimberley, R.C., Harris, C.K., Molnar, J.J., Tomazic, T.J., Eds.; Praeger: Westport, CT, USA, 2002, pp. 87–101.

49. Blackshaw, J.; Blackshaw, A.W. Student perceptions of attitudes to the human animal bond. *Anthrozoös* **1993**, *6*, 190–198.

50. Furnham, A.; Heyes, C. Psychology students' belief about animals and animal experimentation. *Pers. Indiv. Differ.* **1993**, *15*, 1.

51. Paul, E.S.; Serpell, J.A. Childhood pet keeping and humane attitudes in young adulthood. *Anim. Welf.* **1993**, *2*, 321–337.

52. Hagelin, J.; Johansson, B.; Hau, J.; Carlsson, H-E. Influence of pet ownership on opinions toward the use of animals in biomedical research. *Anthrozoös* **2002**, *15*, 251–257.

53. Allport, G.W. *The Nature of Prejudice*; Beacon Press: Cambridge, MA, USA, 1954.

54. Boogaard, B.K.; Oosting, S.J.; Bock, B.B. Elements of societal perception of farm animal welfare: A quantitative study in The Netherlands. *Livest. Sci.* **2006**, *104*, 13–22.

55. Daly, B.; Morton, L.L. An investigation of human-animal interactions and empathy as related to pet preference, ownership, attachment, and attitudes in children. *Anthrozoös* **2006**, *19*, 113–127.

56. Furnham, A.; McManus, C.; Scott, D. Personality, empathy and attitudes to animal welfare. *Anthrozoös* **2003**, *16*, 135–146.

57. Serpell, J.A. *In the Company of Animals: A Study of Human-Animal Relationships*; Cambridge University Press: Cambridge, UK, 1996.

58. Serpell, J.A. Factors influencing human attitudes to animals and their welfare. *Anim. Welf.* **2004**, *13*, S145–S151.

59. Knight, S.; Vrij, A.; Cherryman, J.; Nunkoosing, K. Attitudes towards animal use and animal mind. *Anthrozoös* **2004**, *17*, 43–62.

60. Bowd, A.D.; Bowd, A.C. Attitudes toward the treatment of animals: A study of Christian groups in Australia. *Anthrozoös* **1989**, *3*, 20–24.

61. Forsyth, D.R. A taxonomy of ethical ideologies. *J. Personal. Soc. Psychol.* **1980**, *122*, 175–184.

62. Galvin, S.L.; Herzog, H.A. Ethical ideology, animal right activism and attitudes towards the treatment of animals. *Ethics Behav.* **1992**, *2*, 141–149.

63. Galvin, S.L.; Herzog, H.A. The ethical judgment of animal research. *Ethics Behav.* **1992**, *2*, 263–286.

64. Wuensch, K.; Poteat, G.M. Evaluating the morality of animal research: Effects of ethical ideology, gender, and purpose. *J. Soc. Behav. Personal.* **1998**, *13*, 139–150.

65. Dietz, T.; Frisch, A.S.; Kalof, L.; Stern, P.C.; Guagnano, G.A. Values and vegetarianism: An exploratory analysis. *Rural Sociol.* **1995**, *60*, 533–542.

66. Buss, D.; Craik, K.; Dake, K. Contemporary worldviews and perception of the technological system. In *Risk Evaluation and Management*; Covello, V.T., Menkes, J., Mumpower, J., Eds.; Plenum Press: New York, NY, USA, 1986, pp. 93–130.

67. Herzog, H.A.; Golden, L.L. Moral emotions and social activism: the case of animal rights. *J. Soc. Issues* **2009**, *65*, 485–498.

68. Eurobarometer 55.2. *Europeans, Science and Technology*. 2001. Available online: http://europa.eu.int/comm/research/press/2001/pr0612en_report.pdf (accessed on 25 May 2009).

69. Schuppli, C.A. Decisions about the use of animals in research: Ethical reflection by animal ethics committee members. *Anthrozoös* **2011**, *24*, 409–425.

70. Driscoll, J.W. Attitudes towards animals: Species ratings. *Soc. Anim.* **1995**, *3*, 139–150.

71. Eddy, T.J.; Gallup, G.G.; Povinelli, D.J. Attribution of cognitive states to animals: Anthropomorphism in comparative perspective. *J. Soc. Issues* **1993**, *49*, 87–101.

72. Plous, S. Psychological mechanisms in the human use of animals. *J. Soc. Issues* **1993**, *49*, 11–52.

73. Arluke, A.B. Sacrificial symbolism in animal experimentation: Object or pet? *Anthrozoös* **1988**, *2*, 98–117.

74. Schuppli, C.A.; Fraser, D.; McDonald, M. Expanding the 3Rs to meet new challenges in humane animal experimentation. *Altern. Lab. Anim.* **2004**, *32*, 525–532.

75. Hagelin, J.; Hau, J.; Carlsson, H.E. Attitude of Swedish veterinary and medical students to animal experimentation. *Vet. Rec.* **2000**, *146*, 757–760.

76. Batt, S. Human attitudes towards animals in relation to species similarity to humans: A multivariate approach. *Biosci. Horiz.* **2009**, *2*, 180–190.

77. Gunnthorsdottir, A. Physical attractiveness of a species as a decision factor for its preservation. *Anthrozoös* **2001**, *14*, 204–215.

78. Ormandy, E.H.; Schuppli, C.A; Weary, D.M. Modelling skin cancer in zebrafish or mice: Factors affecting public acceptance. *Altern. Lab. Anim.* **2012**, *40*, 321–333.

79. CCAC. Guidelines on the Care and Use of Fish in Research, Teaching and Testing. 2005. Available online: http://www.ccac.ca/Documents/Standards/Guidelines/Fish.pdf (accessed on 15 March 2014).

80. DeTolla, L.J.; Srinivas, S.; Whitaker, B.R.; Andrews, C.; Hecker, B.; Kane, A.S.; Reimschuessel, R. Guidelines for the care and use of fish in research. *ILAR J.* **1995**, *37*, 159–173.

81. Fabacher, D.L.; Little, E.E. Introduction. In *The Laboratory Fish*; Ostrander, G.K., Ed.; Academic Press: San Diego, CA, USA, 2000; pp. 1–9.

82. Braithwaite, V.A.; Huntingford, F.A. Fish and welfare: Do fish have the capacity for pain perception and suffering? *Anim. Welf.* **2004**, *13*, S87–S92.

83. Chandroo, K.P.; Duncan, I.J.H.; Moccia, R.D. Can fish suffer?: Perspectives on sentience, pain, fear and stress. *Appl. Anim. Behav. Sci.* **2004**, *86*, 225–250.

84. Birke, L.; Arluke, A.; Michael, M. *The Sacrifice: How Scientific Experiments Transform Animals and People*; Purdue University Press: West Lafayette, IN, USA, 2007.

85. Macnaghten, P. *Animal Futures: Public Attitudes and Sensibilities toward Animals and Biotechnology in Contemporary Britain*; IEPPP, Lancaster University: Lancaster, UK, 2001.

86. Rozin, P. The meaning of "natural": Process more important than content. *Psychol. Sci.* **2005**, *16*, 652–658.

87. Midgely, M. Biotechnology and monstrosity: Why we should pay attention to the 'yuk factor'. *Hastings Centre Report* **2000**, *30*, 7–15.

88. Schuppli, C.A.; Molento, C.F.M.; Weary, D.M. Understanding attitudes towards the use of animals in research using an online public engagement tool. *Public Underst. Sci.* **2013.**

89. Macnaghten, P. Animals in their nature: A case study on public attitudes to animals, genetic modification and 'nature'. *Sociology* **2004**, *38*, 533–551.

90. Ormandy, E.H.; Schuppli, C.A.; Weary, D.M. Worldwide trends in the use of animals in research: The contribution of genetically modified animal models. *Altern. Lab. Anim.* **2009**, *37*, 63–68.

91. Aldhous, P.; Coghlan, A.; Copely, J. Let the people speak. *New Sci.* **1999**, *2187*, 26.

92. Henry, B.; Pulcino, R. Individual difference and study-specific characteristics influencing attitudes about the use of animals in medical research. *Soc. Anim.* **2009**, *17*, 305–324.

93. Stanistreet, M. and Spofforth, N. Attitudes of undergraduate students to the uses of animals. *Stud. High. Educ.* **1993**, *18*, 177–196.

94. Richmond, G.; Engelmann, M.; Krupka, L.R. The animal research controversy. *Am. Biol. Teach.* **1990**, *52*, 467–471.

95. Bateson, P. Ethics and behavioral biology. *Adv. Stud. Behav.* **2005**, *35*, 211–233.

96. Morel, V. Causes of the furred and feathered rule the internet. *Nat. Geogr.* 2014. Available online: http://news.nationalgeographic.com/news/2014/03/140314-social-media-animal-rights-groups-animal-testing-animal-cognition-world/?rptregcta=reg_free_np&rptregcampaign=20131016_rw_membership_r1p_intl_ot_w# (accessed on 26 May 2014).

97. Kruse, C.R. The movement and the media: Framing the debate over animal experimentation. *Polit. Commun.* **2001**, *18*, 67–87.

98. Wolch, J.R.; Gullo, A.; Lassiter, U. Changing attitudes towards California's cougars. *Soc. Anim.* **1997**, *5*, 95–116.

99. Sieber, J.E. Students' and scientists' attitudes on animal research. *Am. Biol. Teach.* **1986**, *48*, 85–51.

100. Herzog, H.A.; Dorr, L.B. Electronically available surveys of attitudes toward animals. *Soc. Anim.* **2000**, *8*, 2–8.

101. Kellert, S.R. *Public Attitudes toward Critical Wildlife and Natural Habitat Issues*; PB-80–138332; National Technical Information Service: Springfield, VA, USA, 1980.

102. The Economist. The roar of the crowd: Crowdsourcing is transforming the science of psychology. 2012. Available online: http://www.economist.com/node/21555876 (accessed on 9 May 2013).

103. de Angelis, M.H.; Flaswinkel, H.; Fuchs, H.; Rathkolb, B.; Soewarto, D.; Maschall, S.; Heefner, S.; Pargent, W.; Wuensch, K.; Jung, M.; Reis, A.; Richter, T.; Alessandrini, F.; Jakob, T.; Fuchs, E.; Kolb, H.; Kremmer, E.; Schaeble, K.; Rollinski, B.; Roscher, A.; Peters, C.; Meltinger, T.; Strom, T.; Steckler, T.; Holsboer, F.; Klopstock, T.; Gekeler, F.; Schindewolf, C.; Jung, T.; Avraham, K.; Behrendt, H.; Ring, J.; Zimmer, A.; Schughart, K.; Pfeffer, K.; Wolf, E.; Balling, R. Genome-wide, large-scale production of mutant mice by ENU mutagenesis. *Nat. Genet.* **2000**, *25*, 444–447.

104. de Bruijn, E.; Cuppen, E.; Feitsma, H. Highly efficient ENU mutagenesis in Zebrafish. *Meth. Mol. Biol.* **2010**, *546*, 3–12.

105. Bally, M. University of British Columbia, Vancouver, Canada. Personal communication, 2012.

106. Cummins, R.A.; Gullone, E. Why we should not use 5-point Likert scales: The case for subjective quality of life measurement. In Proceedings of the Second International Conference on Quality of Life in Cities, Singapore, 8–10 March 2000; pp. 79–93.

107. Hobson-West, P. The role of public opinion in the UK animal research debate. *J. Med. Ethics* **2010**, *36*, 46–49.

108. Pytlik Zillig, L.M.; Tomkins, A.J. Public engagement for informing science and technology policy: What do we now, what do we need to know, and how will we get there? *Rev. Policy Res.* **2011**, *28*, 197–217.

109. Kirkwood, J.K.; Hubrecht, R. Animal consciousness, cognition and welfare. *Anim. Welf.* **2001**, *10*, S5–S17.

110. Holmberg, T.; Ideland, M. Secrets and lies: "Selective openness" in the apparatus of animal experimentation. *Public Underst. Sci.* **2012**, *21*, 354–368.

111. Lyons, D. Protecting animals *versus* the pursuit of knowledge: Evolution of the British animal research policy process. *Soc. Anim.* **2011**, *19*, 356–367.

4

Pain Management for Animals Used in Science: Views of Scientists and Veterinarians in Canada

Nicole Fenwick, Shannon E. G. Duffus and Gilly Griffin *

Canadian Council on Animal Care (CCAC), 190 O'Connor St., Suite 800, Ottawa, ON, K2P 2R3, Canada; E-Mails: nfenwick@ccac.ca (N.F.); shannon.duffus@gmail.com (S.E.G.D.)

* Author to whom correspondence should be addressed; E-Mail: ggriffin@ccac.ca.

Simple Summary: Veterinarians, veterinarian-scientists and scientists (all engaged in animal-based studies in Canada) were interviewed to explore the challenges and opportunities for laboratory animal pain management. Our broader aim was to contribute to further discussion of how pain can be minimized for animals used in science. Recognizing when animals are in pain continues to present a challenge, and there does not seem to be consensus on the signs of pain. Clarification of the interactions between scientific objectives and pain management are needed, as well as a stronger evidence base for pain management approaches. Detailed examination of pain management for individual invasive animal models in order to develop model-specific pain management protocols may be useful.

Abstract: To explore the challenges and opportunities for pain management for animals used in research an interview study with 9 veterinarians, 3 veterinarian-scientists and 9 scientists, all engaged in animal-based studies in Canada, was carried out. Our broader aim was to contribute to further discussion of how pain can be minimized for animals used in science. Diverse views were identified regarding the ease of recognizing when animals are in pain and whether animals hide pain. Evidence of inconsistencies in pain management across laboratories, institutions and species were also identified. Clarification of the interactions between scientific objectives and pain management are needed, as well as a stronger evidence base for pain management approaches. Detailed examination of pain management for individual invasive animal models may be useful, and may support the development of model-specific pain management protocols.

Keywords: analgesia; animal models; interview study; pain management; refinement

1. Introduction

The possibility that animals may experience pain when used in science presents an ethical dilemma for both scientists and laboratory animal veterinarians. The dilemma applies both in cases where the pain is a direct consequence of the research (*i.e.*, where pain is the area under study), and in cases where pain is an indirect consequence. The globally accepted ethic of animal experimentation (based on the Three Rs of Russell and Burch [1]) requires that animal pain and distress be minimized (Refinement) [2]. However in some types of animal-based research, pain alleviation measures may be in conflict with scientific objectives. Therefore, concerns regarding the adequacy of pain management continue to be expressed in the scientific literature [3–5].

Some studies have aimed to quantify the prevalence of analgesic administration following surgery and/or other potentially painful procedures in a variety of laboratory animal species [6–9]. The studies concluded that the use of analgesia has increased over time, but the proportion of animals reported as receiving analgesics remains less than the proportion subjected to painful procedures, especially in the case of smaller species [6–9]. Similarly, a Canadian survey of analgesia-withholding found that over 12 months, 42,700 animals (approximately 1.9% of total national use) were used in invasive protocols that received animal ethics committee (AEC) approval to withhold analgesia [10].

Some studies have also identified reasons why analgesia may be withheld or not used. A United Kingdom (UK) survey of scientists and animal care staff found that although respondents had a broad awareness of when there was a potential for animal pain, their accuracy in detecting pain was complicated by a lack of pain indicators and the use of subjective criteria, which may contribute to under-use of analgesia [11]. In the United States (US), a roundtable discussion involving veterinarians, technicians and AEC members identified the lack of knowledge about techniques used to assess, monitor and treat pain as one of the main barriers to reduction of pain in laboratory animals [5]. In the Canadian survey on analgesia-withholding, reasons scientists withheld analgesia included: when analgesia was *proven* conclusively to interfere with experimental results; when analgesia *may* interfere with experimental results; and when pain was part of the phenomenon being studied [10].

To further explore and describe the challenges and opportunities for laboratory animal pain management we undertook a qualitative interview study with veterinarians, veterinarian-scientists and scientists (all engaged in animal-based studies in Canada). Our broader aim is to contribute to further discussion within the scientific community of how pain can be minimized for animals used in science.

2. Methods

A qualitative research approach was selected so that we could elicit and describe the opinions and perspectives of our participants. Using this approach meant that we did not attempt to comprehensively or statistically represent the views of all veterinarians, veterinarian-scientists or animal-based scientists [12]. In addition, our participants are involved in animal-based research in Canada, and therefore it is possible that some of their perspectives and experiences may not resonate with individuals in working in jurisdictions with different animal use oversight mechanisms and/or research environments. To inform our reporting of methodological details we consulted the "consolidated criteria for reporting qualitative research (COREQ)" checklist [13]. Twenty-one interviews were conducted between March and August 2012 (one additional interview was conducted but discarded due to poor quality of the audio recording). Participants included 9 laboratory animal veterinarians (who provided care for animals and had oversight of animal-based research), 3 veterinarian-scientists (who provided care for animals, had oversight of animal-based research and carried out animal-based research) and 9 scientists (who carried out animal-based research). Ethics approval was obtained from Institutional Review Board (IRB) Services (Aurora, ON, Canada) (ICF 111018).

2.1. Participant Selection

Purposive and snowball sampling methods [14] were used to recruit participants who were involved with the use of animals in potentially painful research at Canadian academic institutions. Our initial goal was to recruit participants from each province in Canada (four each from Ontario and Quebec, having the greatest concentration of research institutions and two from each other province). Therefore, an invitation to participate was distributed by email to a listserv of 218 Canadian AEC chairs asking them to distribute the invitation to relevant potential participants. Participant recommendations were also solicited from people known to have an interest in this topic and then invitations to participate were sent via email to the recommended individuals. Subsequently, the participant pool was expanded through referrals from other participants (snowball sampling [14]). We cannot report precisely on the response rate to all our requests for participants because the number of individuals who may have seen the listserv invitation but did not respond is not known. However, five individuals who were contacted directly declined to participate (1 declined outright and 4 initially agreed but then did not respond to subsequent attempts to contact them).

2.2. Participant Demographics

To collect demographic information participants were asked to complete a questionnaire in advance of the interview. Twelve participants were male and 9 were female; 17 participants were current or past members of AECs. Participants' length of professional experience in animal-based science ranged from 5 to 40 years (see Table 1 for experience ranges). Collectively, participants worked in 7 Canadian provinces and 12 different academic institutions. All these institutions had staff veterinarians except for one.

Table 1. Participants' length of professional experience in animal-based science.

	Early Career (<10 years)		Experienced (>10 years)	
	Number of Participants	Years of Experience (Range)	Number of Participants	Years of Experience (Range)
scientists	4	6–9	5	18–40
veterinarians	3	5–10	6	13–22
veterinarian-scientists	1	8	2	20

The 9 scientists and 3 veterinarian-scientists described their research areas as: autoimmune disease, neurobiology, cancer, neuroendocrinology, neurology, neuropharmacology, pain, pharmacology, spinal cord injury, stroke recovery and veterinary medicine. The 9 scientists reported having experience with the following rodent species: mice, rats and gerbils. Participants with veterinary degrees (9 veterinarians, 3 veterinarian-scientists) collectively had experience with a wider range of species including: amphibians, birds, cats, cattle, chinchillas, dogs, ferrets, fish, goats, horses, invertebrates, non-human primates, pigs, sheep, rabbits, reptiles, rodents (including mice, rats and gerbils) and various wild species.

2.3. Interviews

Participants were provided with the study description and consent and confidentiality agreements prior to being interviewed. In the semi-structured interviews participants were asked a series of open-ended questions that had been pilot-tested with the assistance of two veterinarians and one animal-based scientist who were not participants. Interviews, which lasted 1 to 2 h, were conducted face-to-face (7) or by telephone (14) and all were audio-recorded. At the start of each interview, the participant was given a verbal summary of the study and, for face-to-face interviews, asked to sign the consent form. For telephone interviews a signed consent form was obtained in advance. A single investigator carried out all the interviews (SD).

Participants were asked to discuss: (i) procedures and/or animal models they are involved with that may cause pain; (ii) standard drugs and regimes they use to manage pain; (iii) the role of handling and husbandry in pain management; (iv) how an animal in pain is identified; (v) training on recognizing animal pain that is provided at their institution; (vi) how animal pain is monitored; and (vii) what improvements are needed for the management of animal pain. At the end of the interview participants were also asked if there was anything that was not talked about that they considered important. During interviews the term "pain" was used as an umbrella term for stimuli and experiences ranging from a pin prick to severe pain. Participants were not asked to provide a definition of animal pain and the term "animal" was used throughout interviews without necessarily specifying species.

The open-ended style of the interviews allowed participants to respond to each question for as long as they wished and encouraged dialogue, therefore questions were not always delivered in the same order; in many cases participants brought up topics before the question was asked. This format also provided the interviewer with the flexibility to ask follow-up questions, prompted by points brought up by the participant.

2.4. Data Analysis

Interview recordings were transcribed verbatim and numbers were assigned to each participant to anonymize the transcripts. Each transcript was read several times and analysis began with the identification of key concepts and ideas from the text, a process known as coding [15]. Codes were developed both from responses to interview questions and participants' comments that could not be directly related to questions. To develop the coding scheme, two coders (NF and SD) coded the same five interviews and discussed and further refined the coding scheme together. One coder (NF) coded the remaining interviews. The coded sections were then grouped into themes as relationships between codes emerged. In general, our analysis did not attempt to compare the views of one participant group to another as this would not be appropriate with our small, non-statistically representative sample and because not every participant commented on every topic.

To illustrate the research findings, quotations from participants are used, selected on the basis of how well they reflected a given idea and to use quotes from all participants. The quotes have been presented verbatim, although they have been edited to remove interjections (e.g., "um", "uh") and to add punctuation. To provide context for the quotes, they are each ascribed to the participants' role and level of experience (Table 1) and, for veterinarian-scientists and scientists, their self-described research area.

3. Results and Discussion

3.1. Recognizing when Animals are in Pain

3.1.1. Views on Whether Animals are Experiencing Pain Due to Research Use

Some participants readily acknowledged that some animals will unavoidably experience some type of pain as a consequence of scientific use:

> "in terms of animals with, you know, moderate to severe unalleviated pain, I can't think of a project where that would be, you know, the expected outcome. I think there are individual cases, in situations where if people are not effectively assessing or monitoring an animal, that there would be a case where it would experience some pain that was unalleviated" (early career veterinarian)

> "it would be unrealistic to suggest that we could ever not have animals in pain or distress when we use them in research" (experienced veterinarian-scientist studying pharmacology).

Some participants felt that pain in animal-based research is currently well-managed or that anything greater than momentary pain does not occur widely in animal research:

> "most of the time we are able to find something to give some analgesia to the animal ... we don't have really a big problem with that because if it's not possible to give a systemic drug, we at least are able to do local anesthesia" (experienced veterinarian)

> "I tend to believe, and I hope it's not just wishful thinking, but I tend to believe that, or I want to believe that the pain in our procedures is quite minimal" (early career scientist studying neurobiology speaking of his/her own research)

> "if it doesn't hurt, why are we worried?" (experienced pain scientist).

When discussing their local experiences, some study participants perceive that animal pain is well-managed and/or minimal. If this perception was widespread in the animal-based research community then it would be unnecessary to try and draw further attention to unalleviated animal pain and remedy the challenges to animal pain management. In contrast, Canadian and international animal use statistics annually document that animal use does occur at the highest levels of severity, where there is potential for significant pain and distress [16–18].

3.1.2. Ease of Recognizing Pain

Participants held diverse and contradictory views regarding how easily pain can be recognized in laboratory animals. Five of the scientists and one veterinarian expressed confidence that they could readily recognize pain in their own research animals, in part due their knowledge of the individual animals under their care:

> *"either the animals are super, are fine, after two hours all this is normal or they're not and when they're not, they're still in a corner, they're not moving, they're not reacting"* (experienced neuroscientist explaining how s/he determines whether to provide analgesia)

> *"they* [animals] *never seem to hold a grudge against me, you know, the day after a surgery, if, you know, they haven't had buprenorphine* [analgesic drug] *and all that and they seem like they're fine the day after, they don't seem to be upset with me, they come back up to the cage and be interested in playing with me and stuff like normal"* (early career scientist studying stroke).

In contrast, about half of the participants (including veterinarians, veterinarian-scientists and scientists) expressed some uncertainty about their ability to recognize pain and/or felt that recognizing animal pain was difficult:

> *"I don't think he's feeling pain but, you know I'm not, I don't know, I'm not a veterinarian, I don't have that expertise"* (early career neuroscientist recounting the condition of a rodent)

> *"I have no idea if they* [the animals] *are in pain or not, you know, my veterinary training is telling me that probably pain is there but I don't know because I cannot see it, they don't show, either I don't know which behavioral signs will reveal pain or they don't have, they don't show the behavioral signs that will reveal pain, so, that's a problem"* (experienced veterinarian).

Some of the participants who believed that recognizing pain was difficult further commented specifically on the difficulties of recognizing chronic pain:

> *"I'm not sure that I would be able to, truly identify just looking at the animal, if it's kind of a bearable pain"* (experienced veterinarian discussing diagnosis of chronic pain)

> *"the whole issue of chronic pain is very underdiagnosed maybe not diagnosed at all"* (early career veterinarian).

Differing views on whether animals hide their pain were also expressed with some participants believing that animals do hide pain:

> *"it's evolutionarily very important for them to hide pain"* (experienced veterinarian-scientist who studies pharmacology)

> *"the rats are hiding the level of pain, so when you look, subjectively, to* [the] *degree of discomfort and pain, no one was able to detect the rats that were injected with MIA* [painful adjuvant] *and the rats that were injected with saline"* (experienced veterinarian-scientist who studies pain).

Other participants did not support the idea that animals would (or could) hide their pain:

> "*some people have told me that they think that animals hide pain, that's nonsense*" (experienced pain scientist)

> "*we expect that rats will come and run to greet us, if the rat's in pain, they don't do that at all*" (early career stroke scientist)

> "*a rat that's not comfortable will let you know, he or it, I guess, is not comfortable*" (early career neuroendocrinologist)

> "*Oh, they're showing signs, we're just not smart enough to see it*" (early career veterinarian).

To recognize pain, some participants explained how they relied, in part, on their prior experience with animals:

> "*I've worked with them long enough that, that I feel that I can, I can tell, there's certain signs in their facial features, the fur, their behavior, that I'm pretty good, I think, at noticing when something's not right but, again I think it comes with a lot of experience too*" (early career scientist studying neuroendocrinology)

> "*a number of the students that we deal with really don't have any experience with animals of any nature, and so that, in and of itself, creates a very significant challenge*" (experienced veterinarian-scientist who studies pharmacology).

In contrast, just one participant discounted the importance of experience:

> "*there's no way to tell, you know by sitting in front of an individual animal and I just don't buy the fact that there are people that know because they have so much experience*" (experienced pain scientist).

The finding that recognizing animal pain is perceived as challenging is supported by other literature (as discussed in introduction) [4,5,11,19]. It also occurs in other areas of animal use. For example, a 2012 survey of Australian veterinarians' attitudes to providing post-operative analgesia for companion dogs found that 1/5 of respondents did not have confidence in their knowledge of pain and 42% had difficulties recognizing when dogs were experiencing pain [20].

Some participants felt that their experience with animals and pain recognition was helpful for them when making decisions about animal pain management. In contrast, some published research contradicts this view. For example, one study found that experienced observers were no better at detecting pain in rabbits than naive observers [21]. In addition, a review of the usefulness of 'observer ratings' of animal behavior found that although observers with close knowledge of the individual animal are more skilled at observing their behavior, they have a tendency to see positive indicators of welfare in animals that are under their own care [22]. This may contribute to explaining why some participants expressed confidence in their ability to recognize when their own animals were experiencing pain.

3.1.3. Ways of Identifying Pain

Participants reported using a variety of signs to aid in pain recognition including observations of animal behavior and physical appearance, and physiological measurements (e.g., weight, temperature, respiration rate). Participants described using the following behavioral observations: absence of grooming, audible vocalization, decreased social interaction, facial expressions, hunched posture, impaired mobility, lack of nest building (for mice), lethargy, not drinking, over-grooming, place preference (*i.e.,* preference for certain location), reduced appetite, self-mutilation and writhing (for rodents). The following physical signs were described: appearance of masses or bodily secretions, beady eyes (for rodents), coat appearance, dehydration, ocular porphyrin staining (for rodents) and swelling. However, participants also acknowledged these signs can be unreliable and not necessarily indicative of pain:

> *"we don't rely on only one clinical sign to tell us something about the animal, and not every clinical sign is associated with pain, it could be just simply distress or stress"* (experienced veterinarian-scientist studying pharmacology)

> *"we could have something better on there* [pain-scoring checklist] *for specific pain-related things, these are kinda' just general appearance and mobility things that we have on there"* (early career neuroscientist discussing his/her institution's pain-scoring checklist)

> *"with postoperative pain, with any pain stimulus that lasts over about 30 min, you don't get any behavior at all. That's the problem we have"* (experienced pain scientist).

The use of pain-scoring checklists to monitor animals and make decisions about pain alleviation was also discussed and differing views about their usefulness emerged:

> *"we've demanded them from all our, for all protocols submitted to ... our Animal Research Ethics Board. So these humane intervention checkpoints will identify scores which an intervention is provided and they have to, the PIs* [scientists], *have to define that intervention"* (experienced veterinarian-scientist who studies pharmacology)

> *"my first reflex is just not to have to score pain, but just to assume pain is there and to treat it. There's always the question of, if you wait for it, to score it then, by the time you score it, the animal has been in pain for, a few hours"* (experienced veterinarian)

> *"we spent a lot of work, probably for the last 25 years on* [a] *subjective pain scale ... I think it's a loss of time, is not reproducible, is not repeatable and, even not sensitive"* (experienced veterinarian-scientist who studies pain).

About one third of participants commented on how analogies to human experience of similar procedures are used as a way to identify when animals may experience pain:

> *"when in doubt we basically assume it, it's going to hurt, if we think it would hurt us"* (early career veterinarian)

> *"post-operative pain only lasts a few days and, even if we don't know that in mice and rats, we assume it because we know in humans post-operative pain only lasts a couple of days"* (experienced pain scientist).

Guidance documents for using laboratory animals recommend the use of checklists and the identification of clinical signs as a way to determine whether an animal is experiencing pain and distress, and as a tool to determine *a priori* when an experiment should be terminated [23,24]. However, other ways of determining animal pain are now being described in the literature. Examinations of rodent facial expressions and pain-scoring based on expressions has also shown that standard ways of detecting pain can be inaccurate [25–27]. Other research into rodent pain behaviors has shown that signs of pain are more subtle than previously understood [28], and has led to the development of automated pain-detection methods [29,30]. These findings combined with the difficulties of recognizing pain as shown in the literature and acknowledged by some participants in this study, suggest that experience with animals may not be sufficient for reliable pain detection.

3.1.4. Types of Pain

Many participants commented on the difficulties associated with using the term 'pain' as an umbrella term for all painful stimuli and experiences. Some participants felt it would be preferable to correlate the level of concern over pain with its intensity and the animals' ability to "*cope*":

> "*what is more important, is it the pain that we are able to cope with or the pain that we're not able to cope with? Therefore, if you have a chronic pain that you are not able to manage, to cope with you, you will be needing treatment for the pain but if you are able to live with that pain and ... seem to be quite good with it, I mean, is it truly needed to treat that pain?*" (experienced veterinarian using an analogy to the experience of people dealing with a painful condition)

> "*this comes down to a matter of intensity which is something that's lost I think in these discussions, people say the word pain and they're free to, by using the same word, they're free to equalize everything from, you know, the pain of trigeminal neuralgia to a bee sting*" (experienced pain scientist).

These participants felt that this lack of nuance resulted in animal pain being addressed with, inappropriately, 'one-size-fits-all' solutions. They felt that different types of pain should lead to both different levels of concern for animal welfare and different pain management actions. For example, an early career scientist working in stroke research described that the analgesia schedule required to be used at his/her institution was appropriate for a major surgery but not for less invasive procedures. S/he explained that his/her experimental procedures involved creating, "*a small cut and it is on the animal's head but it's not severe in the same way as other surgeries but we've got, we were initially lumped in*" with more invasive procedures. Similarly, another experienced pain scientist commented, "*animal care recommendations don't differentiate between kinds of pain.*"

These comments about different types and intensities of pain suggest that when assessing pain it is important to determine what the animal is actually experiencing (rather than simply assessing, for example, what procedure is performed on the animal) [19,31].

3.2. Pain Management

3.2.1. Approaches to Pain Management

Participants described using both pharmacological and non-pharmacological approaches to alleviating animal pain. Pharmacological approaches included using opioid analgesics, non-steroidal anti-inflammatory drugs (NSAIDs), local and topical anesthetics, as well as general anesthetics during surgery. Many participants reported that they gave groups of animals standardized pain treatment as well as treated animals individually. However, two participants (one veterinarian and one scientist) said they do not provide individualized treatment.

When asked about non-pharmacological pain alleviation strategies, participants described measures related to improving animal comfort, such as softer bedding, lowered lighting and using heat pads or lamps. They also reported lowering water bottles and placing food on the cage floor so that animals in pain would not have to stand and reach for food or water. Changes to food were also mentioned, such as improving nutritional composition, softening food and emphasizing rehydration. Animal handling was mentioned specifically in relation to rodents, including minimizing handling and use of special containers for handling mice, and increasing handling and interaction for rats (although participants did not elaborate on why this may alleviate pain).

Some participants mentioned they use preventative measures such as developing skill in surgical techniques, and ensuring proper techniques are used to administer drugs:

> *"it's quite important to choose the right site, not too close to tail base, then there will be more severe inflammation"* (experienced scientist working on autoimmune diseases describing how injection sites are selected).

Some veterinarians and veterinarian-scientists mentioned defining experimental endpoints as a way to limit and hence manage animal pain. In addition, a few veterinarians also mentioned that occasionally pain alleviation is achieved by presenting scientists with the choice of either providing analgesia or having animal care staff humanely kill an animal prior to conclusion of the experiment.

Participants were asked about what they saw as opportunities to improve pain management for research animals. Some identified technology and the use of automated animal monitoring systems for detecting animals in pain. One participant suggested improving animal nutrition. Others suggested changes related to the use of pharmaceuticals including: improvements to drug formulations so that they are longer acting with longer dosing intervals; use of a greater variety of drugs and drug combinations; routine use of pre-operative medications; and mandatory administration of analgesia and local anesthesia during surgeries.

Other opportunities related to services provided by animal care professionals, such as the use of more animal care staff and centralized animal care and use facilities:

> *"a couple* [of] *really well trained animal techs who could do surgeries for PIs* [scientists], *as opposed to the PI or the graduate student doing the surgery, to ensure that you have better outcomes"* (experienced veterinarian-scientist who studies pharmacology).

The participants in this study described using both pharmacological and non-pharmacological approaches to managing animal pain. Using non-pharmacological measures when analgesics must be withheld is an approach that has been advocated for the refinement of animal models in pain research [4], however, changing the "standard of care" and expectations for the analgesics so that they are universally required (similar to use of anesthetics in surgery) has also been proposed [3,32].

3.2.2. Inconsistencies in Pain Management

Example of inconsistencies in pain management practices across institutions, laboratories and species were mentioned by participants:

"our lab was kinda split between [institution 1] *and* [institution 2] *at the time, we did a study in* [institution 1] *where we had somewhat more lax requirements of what we had to use for analgesia, and we tested, using just a topical, or local anesthetic after surgery, one injection of buprenorphine and then the three injections of buprenorphine used here* [institution 2] *and we saw some effect on the severity of the stroke, in terms of behavioral deficits, as well as an increased mortality in animals that were receiving buprenorphine injections"* (early career stroke scientist describing the different analgesia protocols between two institutions conducting the same research)

"we did that [give analgesics] *at* [previous institution], *we don't do it at* [present institution], *even though I guess we should, and I wouldn't have to ask anyone, I should just do it myself"* (early career scientist studying neuroendocrinology).

Inconsistencies in pain management strategies and resources provided for different species was raised by a few veterinarian participants:

"[in a] large animal operating room, the simple budget of one animal might be, might be 5–10 thousand dollars and in that 5–10 thousand dollars we've got trained animal health technicians, we've got controlled drugs and we're able to do that, whereas in a mouse project, if they're doing 100 mouse surgeries with a graduate student and the budget's smaller, they don't have that, so, so it's a huge issue" (early career veterinarian)

Two veterinarians (one experienced, one early career) commented that pain management options for fish are lacking. Another early career veterinarian commented on how the physical size of the animals affects what can be done for them:

"it's very challenging if not impossible to give an epidural to a mouse or a rat and you can do that for a dog, I think there are some biases because of circumstance that the larger, some of the larger species are probably get more state of the art, if that's what you wanna' term it, analgesia then the rodents do. However I wouldn't, I don't feel in most cases like the rodents are getting insufficient analgesia."

Inconsistencies in analgesia were also attributed by an early career veterinarian (different from above) to difficulties obtaining certain drugs:

"they're not doing it because it takes more effort, it takes more time, some of the drugs are controlled so they have to get their controlled drug license at this institution."

A further example of inconsistency in pain management also emerged when some participants commented on the use of carprofen analgesia in rodent drinking water:

"I've seen tons of SOPs and we have started using it ourselves, putting carprofen in the drinking water of mice prior to doing ear notching and tail amputations, as an attempt at pre-operative anesthesia- or analgesia preemptive analgesia. However we do this knowing there isn't any information out there as to how efficacious it is, how stable it is in water, people have just looked at it anecdotally and a few like, they see some benefit to it and also suggest that they probably aren't doing any harm by doing it" (early career veterinarian)

"we are adamant, you do not put analgesics in the water, you look at the animal and you administer because what happens when you do water is, they're painful they don't drink, they're, 'stuff's in the water', no student comes by to look and to us that's not [an] acceptable form of postoperative monitoring" (early career veterinarian, different from above).

Although our sample was small, a number of inconsistencies in pain management were identified. These inconsistencies have the potential to impact research results as well as the welfare of the animals. However, typically this information is not included in the methods sections of papers that arise from the work, as has been reported in studies that aimed to quantify the prevalence of analgesic administration [6–9]. Use of standardized checklists for reporting methodological details of animal-based research may assist in standardizing this information and decreasing inconsistencies in practice [33].

3.2.3. Pain Management Knowledge

Some scientists described the pain management protocols they used in their research in great detail and complexity with reference to drug mechanisms and pain processes. Others described following the standard or pre-existing protocols at their institution, or the recommendations of the institutional veterinarian:

"when you enter a lab and it's a protocol they've had in place for years, you just kind of accept it and follow it" (early career neuroscientist)

"the procedure that I walked into at [institution], I guess I couldn't really tell you why they chose that" (early career neurobiology scientist commenting on his/her analgesic regime).

This type of situation was also referenced by an early career veterinarian who spoke of pain alleviation protocols as being *"inherited."*

Some veterinarians would prefer that scientists had more knowledge of pain management:

"anesthesia and analgesia are not the same thing and people confuse them so just because you're unconscious does not mean you're free of pain" (early career veterinarian commenting on what s/he perceived as lack of awareness in some scientists)

"I think it's important for them [scientists] to understand the basis for the decisions, and why we make them, and I think if they can understand that they can also understand how some of their actions in surgery might be problematic for an animal in terms of causing excessive amounts of trauma and the inflammation that comes along with it" (early career veterinarian, different from above).

"*in the university, when you're going to work with a PhD that has no experience in medicine* [they] *will be very surprised when you tell them that the animal will receive five or seven, five or six different analgesics, you have to explain a lot*" (experienced veterinarian compared working in a university to a research hospital with medical doctors, who have familiarity with complex analgesic protocols).

Some scientists observed that there is limited evidence-based information to assist in making pain management choices, especially for specific animal models:

"*veterinarians don't even have it* [evidence-based medicine] *because there's simply no evidence base, there're not enough experiments being done, so that there would be any data, you know, to argue about*" (experienced pain scientist comparing the human medicine knowledge base to veterinary medicine)

"*there's a lot of research about, you know, how to manage pain in general and also with all the analgesics, like how effective are these analgesics for different kinds of pain, how long do they last, what kind of doses are effective however, when you start looking into more, specific models ... even just looking at stroke in general, not even the* [specific stroke] *model that we use but, analgesia and stroke, how are these affecting each other, it starts to become a lot more sparse*" (early career scientist studying stroke).

However, some participants felt that research to advance animal pain management knowledge is hampered by lack of resources and/or perceived importance of the work:

"*I think not lots of people participate in these experiments and they need the resource and also what maybe some people will think, it's not so significant a contribution to the science*" (experienced scientist, working on autoimmune diseases)

"*no one's gonna' do it, no one's gonna' pay anybody to do it*" (experienced pain scientist commenting on possible research that could be done to improve pain management for the animal model s/he uses).

"*we all presume that there's pain, I suppose, it's just that, without any evidence of it, it's hard for people to, it's hard for the issue to raise up to the level of priority that it probably deserves*" (experienced pain scientist, different from above)

Participants were in general agreement that there is a lack of scientifically proven information on how to manage animal pain and an absence of resources available to address it. The lack of evidence-based information gives people using animals little option but to make decisions about pain management based on inadequate knowledge. Lack of pain management knowledge, and more specifically lack of scientists' knowledge of pain management were also identified as a barrier to the assessment and treatment of animal pain in a roundtable discussion of laboratory animal professionals (including veterinarians) [5]. It may be useful to clarify what scientists need to know about pain management, and whether it is sufficient for them to collaborate with the institutional veterinarian to devise pain alleviation strategies.

3.3. Pain Management and Research Objectives

Over half of the scientist participants (but no veterinarians or veterinarian-scientists) expressed concern that using analgesia may interfere with their experiments:

"analgesic drugs are powerful drugs that can affect a lot of these processes, so then we get into a situation of where we're using drugs that might interfere" (experienced stroke scientist commenting on the effect of analgesic drugs in stroke recovery)

"we spend a lot of work controlling all that stuff [experimental variables], *now you want me to add a variable? Now that's not good science"* (experienced pain scientist).

One early career scientist studying neuroendocrinology described delaying administration of analgesia due to concern that it would cause excess bleeding:

"I don't want that [analgesia] *to interfere with my study whatsoever so what I do is I give it kinda' half-way through the surgery so it kicks in a little bit later or maybe right after surgery as well and then, I mean, I understand the fact that, you know, the animal will wake up and have a huge headache but it'll have to wait just a little bit until the, my drug will kick in rather than waking up bleeding with no headaches."*

Other scientists and veterinarian-scientists were less concerned about pain control interfering with their research or introducing additional variability:

"I'm a fan, a proponent of variability because if you can see a difference in a system where you know there's a fair bit of biological variability, then I would suggest that whatever intervention, or whatever it is you are doing, that caused that difference between a control and a treatment group ... I'd be more comfortable that that's a real, a real outcome" (experienced veterinarian-scientist who studies pharmacology)

"if there is an effect of the analgesic on the experimental results ... it's an error that we take and accept and it's something that is embedded in all our data, so we may limit the generalization from our data to one lab to another lab but that's typical, so, and besides that, I don't see any limitations ... I worry more about whose doing, running the experiment, it's always a different undergraduate and the data never match, that's more error than giving morphine to the rat" (experienced neuroscientist).

Veterinarians in this study questioned the effect of variability from pain control on experimental outcomes:

"there's no model that's perfect. We're willing to live with the limitations of a model, so why not accept things, that pain control is one of the limitations. That we say, 'okay, well, that's [a] *fact of life' you know. There are things we cannot do with animals and this is one of* [those] *things, we just have to live with it"* (experienced veterinarian)

"no one's ever come back to me and said, 'oh, I could identify those two animals that we treated with analgesia or increased analgesia' ... on their data" (early career veterinarian).

Approximately half of study participants (including veterinarians, veterinarian-scientists and scientists) described how unalleviated pain can interfere with research:

> *"if they're feeling pain they're probably not going to do the tasks that we're hoping to get them to do, since these tasks involve their injured paw ... I would imagine if they're in pain they're not gonna' want to, they either won't do it or, I guess results could be skewed in, you know maybe making it look worse than it actually, their deficit might look worse than it actually is, that kind of thing, so yeah, I think it would definitely have an effect"* (early career neuroscientist who uses behavioral tests in his/her research)

> *"when an animal is in pain, it will induce interference anyway in the process you are studying and this is well known, you have a lot of change induced by the perception of pain and that could affect not only the neuronal system but the hormonal system"* (experienced veterinarian-scientist who studies pain).

Some veterinarians commented on how withholding of analgesia should be justified to AECs:

> *"when I started my practice, it was me who had to prove to them that the analgesic I was prescribing will not affect the study, now it's the contrary, it's them* [scientists] *who have to prove* [to] *the animal care committee* [AEC] *that their, the analgesic, any analgesic will have an impact on their study. So if they say, 'analgesia needs to be withheld', then they will have to provide papers that really say and really show"* (experienced veterinarian)

> *"they* [scientists] *maybe quote some paper that they wrote so I'd say can you send me a copy of that and I'll look it over. We do have, we have had occasion where someone has said we think that this could be impactful, and so we, have said well what we'd like is for you to go ahead and use it* [analgesia] *and then compare that data to previously collected data and see if you can document variance in that data"* (early career veterinarian)

> *"we get a justification for, that this drug can interfere, but we rarely ask the researchers to explain if stress or pain itself can interfere with the, with the project and, also, we tend to forget that there are so many other factors that influence a model and sometimes we kind of stick on this one and forget all the other ones"* (experienced veterinarian, different from above).

In this study, scientist participants raised concerns about pain management interfering with research results, while the veterinarian participants were less concerned. However, participants of all types also commented on how animal pain can impact research results. Assessment of the impact of pain control on research results and the impact of untreated pain on results both suffer from a lack of evidence/information. Efforts to clarify *"what it means to 'affect the model'"* are needed [3] (p. 4) and [19,34].

3.4. Communication, Professional Relationships and Pain Management

Communication, especially between scientists and institutional veterinarians, emerged as an important component of animal pain management. Some veterinarians felt it was important that scientists perceived that they (the veterinarians) understand research, and are not only focused on the animals:

"if you come at them [scientists] *with solely the animal welfare side of things … you know, whether it's pain or distress, environmental enrichment, analgesics, anesthetic, whatever, they tend to either glaze over or dig their heels in. When you come at them with a balanced approach of, you know, 'I'm concerned about your, the robustness of your research model and, you know, by the way, it also ends up, it results in better animal welfare too if we were to do this', then they're far more receptive because they see that you're actually thinking about their research"* (experienced veterinarian)

"[my role is] *being an advocate for the animal…* [but I] *also play a role as a collaborator and a facilitator for a researchers, but a researcher's perspective is often different from my perspective"* (early career veterinarian).

Some scientists commented on how it was useful for them to pro-actively communicate with their institutional veterinarian:

"we communicated [with] *each other and discussed the procedure, so I think it's quite, it's quite helpful for them* [veterinarians] *to understand why we have to do this and also why we should not give the mice any analgesia"* (experienced scientist studying autoimmune diseases)

"for my purposes, and if the vet tells me that it's [a pain treatment] *more appropriate, I'm gonna' go with her judgment, of course and my animals look great"* (experienced neuroscientist describing trusting the expertise of their institution's veterinarian).

Many veterinarians spoke about relying on their past experience with the individuals conducting the research when it came to checking compliance with analgesia administration:

"we tend to know also the team who is working, so depending on the team we can have, additional monitoring of the animal if we feel that we're not certain that they're giving the analgesic properly" (experienced veterinarian)

"there's less involvement, obviously with the more experienced labs … we kind of leave it up to them, to let us know if it's working or not" (early career veterinarian).

A few veterinarians (but no scientists) also described acting more assertively to mitigate pain. For example, an experienced veterinarian attributed the success s/he had in making changes to institutional analgesic routines, *"partly because I push a lot,"* while an early career veterinarian explained how s/he responded sometimes in situations where a scientist has been reluctant to provide supportive treatment to a sick animal:

"you can't warm it up, you can't give it fluids, you can't give it analgesics, then we're gonna' say okay we're gonna' kill it."

The importance of professional communication also emerged when participants spoke about other workers in research laboratories. For example, an early career veterinarian expressed concern with the turnover in laboratory personnel and the lack of communication that can occur:

"in the rush to get a lot of work done and people, you know, summer students or grad students coming in and out of labs, there's not really a lot of communication, everyone's busy so they don't necessarily discuss the fine, fine details of, you know, detecting pain in animals, what's indicative of, you know appropriate pain management or not."

This participant also linked the success of pain alleviation to communication, worrying that steps described in an animal care protocol may not be implemented if there is a lack of communication. An early career scientist in neurobiology described how poor communication could also affect research objectives:

"sometimes the [animal care] staff and what they want done can interfere with what needs to be done in the lab and so, sometimes you have to come to some kind of agreement as to, okay what drugs are we gonna' use that manages pain enough but also doesn't interfere with the studies that we're trying to do."

Participants in this study described the usefulness of communication between the professionals engaged in animal-based research. Building on this strength, workshops and more formalized collaborations could seek to resolve questions regarding the respective roles of scientists and veterinarians in animal pain management, an approach that has also been proposed to improve professional communications about laboratory animal environments [35].

4. Conclusions

This study aimed to explore and describe the challenges and opportunities for pain management for animals used in science and, through this, contribute to discussions of how pain can be minimized. Previous research [6–9] has shown that that the use of analgesia for pain management of animals used in science has increased over time, but the proportion of animals reported as receiving analgesics remains less than the proportion subjected to painful procedures. Other survey and workshop studies identified some reasons why analgesia may be withheld or not used, such as lack of pain indicators, lack of knowledge about techniques used to assess, monitor and treat pain and when analgesia is proven or believed to interfere with experimental results [5,10,11]. The interview methodology of the present study has elaborated on these reasons and provided additional possible reasons for the gap between animal pain and pain management.

When speaking of their local experiences some participants in this study perceived that animal pain is well-managed and/or minimal, in contrast to concerns regarding the overall adequacy of pain management in animal-based science expressed in other literature [3–5] and animal use statistics that document animal use at high severity levels [16–18]. Similar to other studies for example, [5,11,28], we also found that recognizing when, and to what degree, animals are in pain continues to present challenges, in part because there does not seem to be consensus on the signs of pain.

A number of inconsistencies in pain management practices across institutions, laboratories and species that have the potential to impact research results and animal welfare were described by participants. However, typically this type of information is not included in the methods sections of papers that arise from the work, as has been reported in studies that aimed to quantify the prevalence of analgesic administration [6–9].

Participants were in general agreement that there is a lack of scientifically proven information on how to manage animal pain and an absence of resources available to address it, similar to the findings of other studies [5,10,11,28]. This suggests that clarification of the interactions between scientific objectives and pain management is needed, as well as a stronger evidence base for pain management approaches, as has also been proposed by other authors [28,36]. Animal pain management may be best addressed by discipline and/or model-specific research, considering the vastness of different conditions and circumstances of each research area. Detailed examinations of existing pain management protocols for individual animal models leading to development of standardized model-specific pain protocols may be a useful approach. Similarly, a review of behavior measurements of pain in rodents concluded that assessment of chronic pain likely needs to be procedure and species specific [28]. Model-specific protocols may be readily adopted by scientists, as it emerged that some scientists in this study willingly following established protocols at their institution.

Acknowledgments

The authors gratefully acknowledge: individuals who generously shared their time as participants in this study; Elisabeth Ormandy for comments on an earlier version of this paper; and the valuable feedback from three anonymous reviewers. Funding for this study was provided by the CCAC Fellowship program.

Author Contributions

Nicole Fenwick analyzed the data and wrote the paper. Shannon Duffus conceived and co-designed the study, collected all data, participated in coding and provided revisions to drafts of the paper. Gilly Griffin supervised and co-designed the study and provided revisions to drafts of the paper.

Conflicts of Interest

Funding for this study was provided by the Canadian Council on Animal Care (CCAC) Fellowship Program. The authors are current (NF, GG) and past (SG) employees of CCAC.

References

1. Russell, W.; Burch, R. *The Principles of Humane Experimental Technique*; Unversities Federation for Animal Welfare: Potters Bar, UK, 1959; p. 238.

2. Fenwick, N.; Griffin, G.; Gauthier, C. The welfare of animals used in science: How the "Three Rs" ethic guides improvements. *Can. Vet. J.* **2009**, *50*, 1–8.

3. Carbone, L. Pain in laboratory animals: The ethical and regulatory imperatives. *PLoS ONE* **2011**, *6*.

4. Magalhães-Sant'Ana, M.; Sandøe, P.; Olsson, I.A.S. Painful dilemmas : The ethics of animal-based pain research. *Anim. Welf.* **2009**, *18*, 49–63.

5. Karas, A.Z. Barriers to assessment and treatment of pain in laboratory animals. *Lab Anim. (NY)* **2006**, *35*, 38–45.

6.   Coulter, C.A.; Flecknell, P.A.; Richardson, C.A. Reported analgesic administration to rabbits, pigs, sheep, dogs and non-human primates undergoing experimental surgical procedures. *Lab. Anim.* **2009**, *43*, 232–238.

7.   Coulter, C.A.; Flecknell, P.A.; Leach, M.C.; Richardson, C.A. Reported analgesic administration to rabbits undergoing experimental surgical procedures. *BMC Vet. Res.* **2011**, *7*, doi:10.1186/1746-6148-7-12.

8.   Richardson, C.A.; Flecknell, P.A. Anaesthesia and post-operative analgesia following experimental surgery in laboratory rodents : are we making progress ? *Altern. Lab. Anim.* **2005**, *33*, 119–127.

9.   Stokes, E.L.; Flecknell, P.A.; Richardson, C.A. Reported analgesic and anaesthetic administration to rodents undergoing experimental surgical procedures. *Lab. Anim.* **2009**, *43*, 149–154.

10. Fenwick, N.; Tellier, C.; Griffin, G. *The Characteristics of Analgesia-Withholding in Animal-Based Scientific Protocols in Canada*; Canadian Council on Animal Care (CCAC): Ottawa, ON, Canada, 2010.

11. Hawkins, P. Recognizing and assessing pain, suffering and distress in laboratory animals: A survey of current practice in the UK with recommendations. *Lab. Anim.* **2002**, *36*, 378–395.

12. Silverman, D. *Doing Qualitative Research*; SAGE Publications: Thousand Oaks, CA, USA, 2000; p. 316.

13. Tong, A.; Sainsbury, P.; Craig, J. Consolidated criteria for reporting qualitative research (COREQ): A 32-item checklist for interviews and focus groups. *Int. J. Qual. Heal. Care* **2007**, *19*, 349–357.

14. Palys, T.; Atchison, C. Sampling. In *Research Decisions: Quantitative and Qualitative Perspectives*; Veitch, E., Ed.; Nelson Education Ltd.: Toronto, ON, Canada, 2007; pp. 107–135.

15. Coffey, A.; Atkinson, P. Concepts and coding. In *Making Sense of Qualitative Data: Complementary Research Strategies*; Coffey, A.; Atkinson, P., Eds.; SAGE Publications: Thousand Oaks, CA, USA, 1996; pp. 26–53.

16. Canadian Council on Animal Care (CCAC). Animal Use Data for 2011. Available online: http://ccac.ca/en_/publications/audf/stats-aud/data-2011 (accessed on 14 May 2014).

17. Home Office. Annual Statistics of Scientific Procedures on Living Animals, Great Britain 2012. Available online: https://www.gov.uk/government/publications/statistics-of-scientific-procedures-on-living-animals-great-britain-2012 (accessed on 14 May 2014).

18. European Commission. Animals Used for Scientific Purposes. Statistical Reports. Available online: http://ec.europa.eu/environment/chemicals/lab_animals/reports_en.htm (accessed on 14 May 2014).

19. *Recognition and Alleviation of Pain in Laboratory Animals*; National Research Council (US) Committee on Recognition and Alleviation of Pain in Laboratory Animals: Washington, DC, USA, 2009.

20. Weber, G.H.; Morton, J.M.; Keates, H. Postoperative pain and perioperative analgesic administration in dogs: Practices, attitudes and beliefs of Queensland veterinarians. *Aust. Vet. J.* **2012**, *90*, 186–193.

21. Leach, M.C.; Coulter, C.A.; Richardson, C.A.; Flecknell, P.A. Are we looking in the wrong place? Implications for behavioral-based pain assessment in rabbits (Oryctolagus cuniculi) and beyond? *PLoS ONE* **2011**, *6*, e13347.

22. Meagher, R.K. Observer ratings: Validity and value as a tool for animal welfare research. *Appl. Anim. Behav. Sci.* **2009**, *119*, 1–14.

23. *CCAC Guidelines on: Choosing an Appropriate Endpoint in Experiments Using Animals for Research, Teaching and Testing*; Canadian Council on Animal Care (CCAC): Ottawa, ON, Canada, 1998.

24. *OECD Guidance Document on the Recognition, Assessment, and Use of Clinical Signs as Humane Endpoints for Experimental Animals Used in Safety Evaluation*; Organization for Economic Cooperation and Development (OECD): Paris, France, 2000.

25. Sotocinal, S.G.; Sorge, R.E.; Zaloum, A.; Tuttle, A.H.; Martin, L.J.; Wieskopf, J.S.; Mapplebeck, J.C.S.; Wei, P.; Zhan, S.; Zhang, S.; *et al.* The Rat Grimace Scale: A partially automated method for quantifying pain in the laboratory rat via facial expressions. *Mol. Pain* **2011**, *7*, 55.

26. Matsumiya, L.C.; Sorge, R.E.; Sotocinal, S.G.; Tabaka, J.M.; Wieskopf, J.S.; Zaloum, A.; King, O.D.; Mogil, J.S. Using the Mouse Grimace Scale to reevaluate the efficacy of postoperative analgesics in laboratory mice. *J. Am. Assoc. Lab. Anim. Sci.* **2012**, *51*, 42–49.

27. Langford, D.J.; Bailey, A.L.; Chanda, M.L.; Clarke, S.E.; Drummond, T.E.; Echols, S.; Glick, S.; Ingrao, J.; Klassen-Ross, T.; Lacroix-Fralish, M.L.; *et al.* Coding of facial expressions of pain in the laboratory mouse. *Nat. Methods* **2010**, *7*, 447–449.

28. Whittaker, A.L.; Howarth, G.S. Use of spontaneous behavior measures to assess pain in laboratory rats and mice: How are we progressing? *Appl. Anim. Behav. Sci.* **2014**, *151*, 1–12.

29. Roughan, J.V.; Wright-Williams, S.L.; Flecknell, P.A. Automated analysis of postoperative behavior: Assessment of HomeCageScan as a novel method to rapidly identify pain and analgesic effects in mice. *Lab. Anim.* **2009**, *43*, 17–26.

30. Wright-Williams, S.; Flecknell, P.A.; Roughan, J.V. Comparative effects of vasectomy surgery and buprenorphine treatment on faecal corticosterone concentrations and behavior assessed by manual and automated analysis methods in C57 and C3H mice. *PLoS ONE* **2013**, *8*, e75948.

31. Honess, P.; Wolfensohn, S. The extended welfare assessment grid: A matrix for the assessment of welfare and cumulative suffering in experimental animals. *Altern. Lab. Anim.* **2010**, *38*, 205–212.

32. McKeon, G.; Pacharinsak, C.; Long, C.; Howard, A.; Jampachaisri, K.; Yeomans, D.; Felt, S. Analgesic Effects of Tramadol, Tramadol–Gabapentin, and Buprenorphine in an Incisional Model of Pain in Rats (*Rattus norvegicus*). *J. Am. Assoc. Lab. Anim. Sci.* **2011**, *50*, 192–197.

33. Kilkenny, C.; Browne, W.J.; Cuthill, I.C.; Emerson, M.; Altman, D.G. Improving bioscience research reporting: The ARRIVE guidelines for reporting animal research. *PLoS Biol.* **2010**, *8*, e1000412.

34. Percie du Sert, N.; Rice, A.S.C. Improving the translation of analgesic drugs to the clinic: Animal models of neuropathic pain. *Br. J. Pharmacol.* **2014**, *171*, 2951–2963.

35. Baumans, V.; Van Loo, P. How to improve housing conditions of laboratory animals: The possibilities of environmental refinement. *Vet. J.* **2013**, *195*, 24–32.

36. Hubrecht, R. *The Welfare of Animals Used in Research*; Wiley Blackwell: Wheathampstead, UK, 2014; p. 271.

5

The Mississippi State University College of Veterinary Medicine Shelter Program

Philip Bushby *, Kimberly Woodruff and Jake Shivley

College of Veterinary Medicine, Mississippi State University, P.O. Box 6001, Mississippi State, MS 39762, USA; E-Mails: kwoodruff@cvm.msstate.edu (K.W.); jshivley@cvm.msstate.edu (J.S.)

* Author to whom correspondence should be addressed; E-Mail: bushby@cvm.msstate.edu.

Academic Editor: Marina von Keyserlingk

Simple Summary: First initiated in 1995 to provide veterinary students with spay/neuter experience, the shelter program at the Mississippi State University College of Veterinary Medicine has grown to be comprehensive in nature incorporating spay/neuter, basic wellness care, diagnostics, medical management, disease control, shelter management and biosecurity. Junior veterinary students spend five days in shelters; senior veterinary students spend 2-weeks visiting shelters in mobile veterinary units. The program has three primary components: spay/neuter, shelter medical days and Animals in Focus. Student gain significant hands-on experience and evaluations of the program by students are overwhelmingly positive.

Abstract: The shelter program at the Mississippi State University College of Veterinary Medicine provides veterinary students with extensive experience in shelter animal care including spay/neuter, basic wellness care, diagnostics, medical management, disease control, shelter management and biosecurity. Students spend five days at shelters in the junior year of the curriculum and two weeks working on mobile veterinary units in their senior year. The program helps meet accreditation standards of the American Veterinary Medical Association's Council on Education that require students to have hands-on experience and is in keeping with recommendations from the North American Veterinary Medical Education Consortium. The program responds, in part, to the challenge from the Pew Study on Future Directions for Veterinary Medicine that argued that veterinary students do not graduate with the level of knowledge and skills that is commensurate with the number of years of professional education.

Keywords: Surgical instruction; animal shelter; shelter medicine; spay/neuter; shelter education; shelter management; veterinary education

---

1. Introduction

The American Veterinary Medical Association (AVMA) Council on Education (COE) requires veterinary schools to "provide instruction in both the theory and practice of medicine and surgery." The accreditation standards for veterinary colleges state that "must include principles and hands-on experiences in physical and laboratory diagnostic methods and interpretation, … disease prevention, biosecurity, therapeutic intervention (including surgery)" among several other skills [1] The recent study by the North American Veterinary Medical Educational Consortium (NAVMEC) concluded "to achieve entry-level competency, students should be provided sufficient time and opportunity to learn and practice necessary knowledge and skills [2]." It is, therefore, clear that one of the expectations of a veterinary curriculum is to provide students with ample hands-on practical experience. Yet the Pew National Veterinary Education Program's study entitled Future Directions for Veterinary Medicine concluded, in part, that "veterinary graduates, with few exceptions, have been unable to acquire the level of knowledge and skills which should be achieved, considering the many years devoted to a professional veterinary education [3]."

In 1995, in an effort to increase the hands-on clinical experience of veterinary students the College of Veterinary Medicine at Mississippi State University developed a cooperative program with a local animal shelter. Over the years the shelter program has grown in stages. Early on the program focused on spay/neuter surgery. From 1995 to 2007 the program was limited to one or two local shelters that had their own surgical suite. In 2007, the College obtained a mobile veterinary unit. No longer limited to shelters with a surgical suite the program rapidly grew to serve 14 different animal shelters. In 2013, with the addition of a second mobile veterinary unit the program expanded to 20 animal shelters and enrollment was opened as an extern experience for students from other veterinary schools. In 2014 the program was expanded to include an increased emphasis on shelter animal wellness care, medical management and shelter management as well as developing an educational component that targets elementary school children.

2. Program Development

2.1. The Early Years, 1995 to 2007

During the early years the shelter program at the Mississippi State University College of Veterinary Medicine involved just third year veterinary students. Third year students have nine months of clinical activities in the veterinary teaching hospital. This includes a 6-week primary care rotation focused on routine small animal care. Initially every student in the primary care rotation spent one day at a local animal shelter performing spays and neuters under the supervision of a board certified surgeon. Students took turns rotating though the surgical suite performing surgeries with a faculty surgeon scrubbed in as their assistant. The role of the faculty member was to guide the student through the procedures, intervene to prevent errors, help the students when there were problems, and provide verbal and written feedback to the students after the surgeries were completed.

Conducted as a "mash style" spay/neuter activity, all necessary surgical supplies were transported to the shelter along with the students and faculty member. The shelter provided the surgical suite, surgical table, anesthetic machine and, of course, the animals. Shelter personnel would select the animals they wished to present for surgery. Pending the results of a brief physical examination, patients would be anesthetized, prepped for surgery and transported to the surgical suite one at a time. Cases were assigned to give each student equal opportunity to perform each of the surgical procedures; cat spay, cat castration, dog spay, and dog castration.

Initially all surgeries were performed on adult (over 6 months old) dogs and cats. Shelter management resisted the practice of early age or pediatric spay/neuter in spite of the fact that a majority of adoptions were puppies and kittens. Eventually, with a change in shelter management, pediatric spay/neuter was added to the program thereby providing students with experience in performing spays and neuters of puppies and kittens as young as six to eight weeks of age.

In 2005 the shelter program doubled in size. When a local humane society built a new animal shelter that included a surgical suite, the college expanded the program to include that shelter. Rather than reduce the trips to the original shelter the approach was to simply add more trips. With this addition every third year student spent 2 days (one in each of the two shelters) performing spays and neuters.

2.2. Mobile Veterinary Units

The College obtained its first mobile veterinary unit as a result of Hurricane Katrina. In 2005, Hurricane Katrina created massive destruction on the Mississippi and Louisiana gulf coast. One of the aftermaths of Hurricane Katrina was an increase in funding for animal rescue and spay/neuter along the gulf coast. A grant from the American Kennel Club Companion Area Recovery along with private donations allowed for the purchase of a mobile veterinary unit designed for disaster recovery and spay/neuter (See Figure 1). A grant from the Humane Society of the United States provided funding to expand the shelter program and operate the mobile unit.

With the acquisition of the mobile unit the college was no longer limited to shelters that had their own surgical suite, so the program rapidly expanded to 14 shelters. The college created a senior year shelter medicine spay/neuter elective rotation. The 2-week rotation functioned year round except for Christmas and New Year's break and could enroll two senior students at a time. Shelters would still select their patients, but with the mobile unit the program was no longer limited to just one surgery being performed at a time. The junior students still made two trips to shelters and still scrubbed in with a faculty member acting as assistant. Junior students averaged 15 sterilization surgeries in those two trips. Up to 50 senior students could enroll in the elective each year. Senior students would make seven or eight trips to shelters. On the first day of the 2-week elective a faculty member would scrub in with the senior students for each surgery, but after that first day senior students performed the surgeries unassisted. A faculty member or resident was always supervising surgeries and could scrub in to assist if necessary, but for the most part students performed the surgeries on their own. As long as the safety of the patient was not at risk, students were given the chance to handle problems/complications on their own. Senior students would average over 70 surgeries each during the 2-week rotation. With this many surgeries in a concentrated period of time, most students became efficient and confident in their surgical skills.

The program still had limited enrollment during this period. Enrolling two students for 2-weeks at a time, 50 weeks of the year, kept enrollment at 50 students a year. Demand for the elective was great but with a class size of 80 to 85 students per year approximately 40% of each senior class was unable to enroll. Discontented with the situation, the freshmen Class of 2014 initiated a project to raise funds to purchase a second mobile unit. When PetSmart Charities heard of the students efforts they funded a grant to purchase a second mobile unit (See Figure 2).

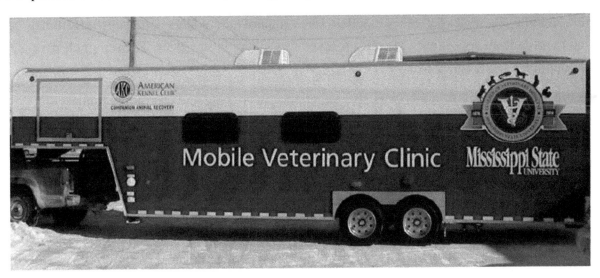

Figure 1. Mississippi State University College of Veterinary Medicine's first mobile unit. Mississippi State University College of Veterinary Medicine's first mobile unit is a 32 ft gooseneck trailer fully equipped for spay/neuter of dogs and cats at animal shelters

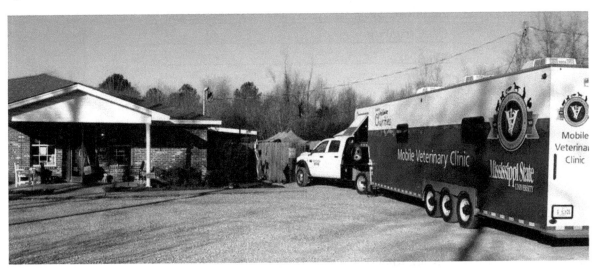

Figure 2. Mississippi State University College of Veterinary Medicine's second mobile unit at a local animal shelter. Mississippi State University College of Veterinary Medicine's second mobile unit is a 38 ft gooseneck trailer equipped with three surgical tables for performing spays and neuters

The second mobile unit was put into service in January of 2013, just in time for the Class of 2014 to be the first class in which every student who wished to take the Shelter elective could enroll. Every junior student still goes on two trips, but the capacity for senior students expanded from 50 to 120. With an enrollment of 85 students per class at Mississippi State University College of Veterinary Medicine there is room to enroll between 35 and 40 senior students from other schools in the elective. The 2-week elective is offered 48 weeks per year and can accommodate five senior students each rotation. Each mobile unit goes to seven or eight different shelters during the 2-week rotation and senior students still average nearly 70 surgeries each.

2.3. Learning Resources

The intent of the junior experience at shelters is to acquaint the students with the issues animal shelters face and to provide an opportunity to perform several sterilization surgeries. The senior elective is much more in-depth and is designed to:

- Provide veterinary students extensive experience in spaying and castrating animals that will be placed for adoption;
- Provide veterinary students with first-hand experience in dealing with the medical behavioral and surgical problems encountered in animals confined to animal shelters;
- Increase veterinary students' understanding of the issues surrounding overpopulation of unwanted pets;
- Prepare veterinary students to work closely with local humane societies and animal shelters to find solutions to the overpopulation of unwanted pets in the local community.

Table 1. Surgical Instructional Videos. Students review videos of all surgical techniques and procedures prior to performing surgery on the mobile veterinary units.

Adult Dog Castration
Adult Dog Spay
Cat Castration
Cat Spay
Closure
Cryptorchid (Abdominal—Spay Hook technique)
Cryptorchid (Abdominal—under bladder technique)
Cryptorchid (Subcutaneous)
Flank Spay
Millers Knot (Hand tie)
Pedicle Tie
Puppy Castration
Puppy Spay
Square Knot (Hand tie)
Surgeons Knot (Hand tie)
Born to Die

The surgical techniques used are similar to those used in high volume spay/neuter clinics and are consistent with the standards outlined by the Association of Shelter Veterinarians (ASV). (REF) All students who participate in the program are required to view videos of the surgical techniques prior to performing surgery (See table 1).

Understanding of these surgical techniques is then reinforced by the faculty who scrub in to assist the juniors on both days that they perform surgery and for seniors and extern students on the first day of their rotation.

Senior students and externs in the 2-week elective are given assigned reading to increase their understanding of the problems associated with over-population of unwanted dogs and cats, the standards of care in spay/neuter clinics, and standards of care in animal shelters (See Table 2).

Table 2. Assigned Reading. Reading assignments in advance of the shelter elective prepare students to understand the issues that animal shelters routinely face.

Guidelines for Standards of Care in Animal Shelters [4]
The Association of Shelter Veterinarians Veterinary Medical Care Guidelines for Spay-Neuter Programs [5]
How Could You [6]
PTS [7]
Letter from a Shelter Manager [8]

2.4. Impact of the Spay Neuter Program

The program has an impact both on the veterinary students and on the shelters that participate. Since the inception of the program over 55,000 sterilization surgeries have been performed at local shelters. Since the first mobile unit was acquired in 2007, over 51,000 surgeries have been performed. The adoption rate of the animals that have been sterilized are extremely high, even in shelters that have high euthanasia rates. The program has clearly saved the lives of numerous animals by increasing the adoption rates (in 2013 collectively the euthanasia rate of the shelters we work with was 62%, but the adoption rate of the animals sterilized in our program was 82%). Furthermore, the animals adopted are sterilized preventing future litters of puppies and kittens, and for some shelters reducing the intake numbers over time.

The increased surgical skills and understanding of the problems of pet overpopulation by the veterinary students is, however, the true impact. Students learn high quality high volume spay/neuter techniques in both pediatric and adult dogs and cats. On average each student performs 67 sterilizations during his/her 2-week rotation, See Table 3). Doing this many surgeries in a 2-week period increases student skill, efficiency and confidence. Allowing students to work through surgical difficulties and complications also builds their confidence.

Table 3. Average number of surgeries of each type performed by senior veterinary students.

	kitten neuter	cat neuter	kitten spay	cat spay	puppy neuter	dog neuter	puppy spay	dog spay	Total
Average per student	5	7	9	8	6	10	11	10	67

Veterinary students participating in the shelter elective at Mississippi State University College of Veterinary Medicine gain extensive surgical experience performing spays and castrations of adult and pediatric dogs and cats.

Students are overwhelmingly positive about the experience. Senior students in the 2-week elective consistently rate the experience as one of the most valuable in their veterinary education.

Student evaluations of the shelter elective at Mississippi State University College of Veterinary Medicine are consistently very positive (See Tables 4 and 5).

Table 4. Student evaluations of the shelter elective since acquisition of the second mobile unit.

	Number of Students Responding						
	Strongly Disagree	Disagree	Neutral	Agree	Strongly Agree	Total Number	Mean on 5 pt. score
The rotation met my expectations	2	0	2	22	158	184	4.82
Participating in the Mobile Spay Neuter trips was valuable	2	0	3	12	167	184	4.86
The assigned articles were valuable	2	1	21	53	107	184	4.42
The rotation gave me an understanding of the issues surrounding overpopulation of unwanted pets	2	0	4	32	146	184	4.74
The rotation gave me increased experience in spaying and castrating animals	2	0	3	8	171	184	4.88
I would recommend this elective to others	2	0	2	11	169	184	4.88
The videos of surgical procedures helped prepare me for the course	2	1	4	23	154	184	4.77

Table 5. Typical comments from senior veterinary students.

It was a great experience and I appreciate all the patience and great teaching skills.
I loved this rotation. This was a great rotation to allow the students to have more freedom to improve their surgical skills but to have a doctor there to help with any questions/problems we could encounter. I would absolutely recommend this rotation to others.
I was able to improve my surgical skills and better my understanding of shelter management and current issues.
Great rotation and very valuable surgical experience!
I was able to improve my surgical skills and better my understanding of shelter management and current issues.
This is an amazing elective. I was able to learn a lot and refine my skills and efficiency. The doctors and technicians were fantastic to work with. They were very patient and willing to help out a lot in any situation. This is a very valuable elective.
I did appreciate that I was allowed to manage my own surgical complications; that definitely helped improve my surgical competency and confidence level for managing complications.
This was the most valuable rotation that I have participated in during my vet school experience. I have a strong interest in surgery and feel that my surgical skills have greatly improved due to this experience.

Students appreciate the opportunity to gain extensive surgical experience during the shelter elective at the Mississippi State University College of Veterinary Medicine.

Extern students frequently provide feedback as well: "This rotation is extremely valuable to my education. At my school we only get one spay and one neuter prior to graduation, which is why I came here. You guys have made me much more comfortable in surgery. For that I am so grateful."

With the elective receiving such positive reviews and with the addition of the second mobile unit enrollment in the course has steadily increased over time (See Table 6).

Table 6. Student enrollment. Student enrollment in the shelter elective at Mississippi State University College of Veterinary Medicine has increased consistently since the inception of the program in 2007.

Academic year	Number of Students Enrolled
2007 *	6
2007–2008	37
2008–2009	35
2009–2010	41
2010–2011	48
2011–2012	48
2012–2013 **	70
2013–2014	106
2014–2015 ***	92

*: Rotation began spring semester 2007; **: 2nd Mobile Unit put into operation January 2013; ***: At time of submission this number represents only about 80% of the year

3. Program Expansion

3.1. Shelter Medical Days

In May of 2013, a second component Shelter Medical Days was added to the program expanding the emphasis from spay/neuter and animal wellness to include shelter disease control and biosecurity. Shelter medical days are currently housed within the 6-week Community Veterinary Services junior rotation. Each student spends at least 3 days of the rotation at an animal shelter in the surrounding area, increasing the number of days spent in a shelter from 2 days on the mobile unit to a total of 5 days. Typically, a shelter medical day begins with a biosecurity walk-through of the shelter. In order to encourage students to look critically at breaks in biosecurity, they are given the task of completing a "photo scavenger hunt". To complete the scavenger hunt they must take pictures of breaks in biosecurity, of good biosecurity practices, and signs of disease. The only rules are that all of the pictures must be taken on the camera belonging to the shelter medicine program and no employee faces can be in the photos. After all of the students have completed their 3 shelter medical days, the pictures are collated and discussed during a grand rounds session. Discussion includes explanations of why the picture was taken as well as what should be done to correct any breaks in biosecurity or prevent any transmission of disease.

Following the walk through at the shelter, students spend the remainder of the shelter medical day performing physicals, basic diagnostic tests and behavior assessments. Students have access to supplies for basic fecal floats, cytology, skin scrapes or any other easily transportable tests. Students also have access to ophthalmoscopes, otoscopes, and stethoscopes. Under the supervision of a faculty member students perform exams, diagnostic tests and make diagnosis and treatment plans for the animals in the care of the shelter.

Shelter Medical Days give all junior veterinary students experience in routine physical examinations and routine diagnostics. Students encounter conditions that are not commonly presented to the veterinary teaching hospital, but are commonly encountered in private veterinary practice. In addition, this program provides students with an increased understanding of disease control, disease prevention and biosecurity in the shelter environment.

3.2. Animals in Focus

In 2014, a third arm, Animals in Focus (AIF), was added to the shelter program. AIF is an elementary school program direct at children in socioeconomically disadvantaged areas in Mississippi. In these areas animal neglect and abuse, such as dog fighting, tend to be more prevalent than in some other areas of the state. The intent of this program is to introduce students to the needs of animals, increase the perceived value of animal life, and to use animals as a teaching tool for individual health of both the pet and the children. AIF uses fun and interactive programs to establish relationships with the students and teachers in the schools. An imperative part of the program is using animals (most often dogs) as teachers. The children play games with the animals, learn how to safely interact with animals, and begin to place a higher value on the lives of animals in general. In addition, the hope is that teachers are able to use pets as teaching tools in the classroom. The expectation is that this will increase enthusiasm in the classroom, improve attendance, and generate higher levels of self-confidence in the students.

While AIF is a great program for children in these areas across the state, it is a benefit for the veterinary students as well. Veterinary students in their third year are invited to volunteer for AIF trips. Generally, 4–5 students participate in each trip. These trips are in addition to the junior year spay neuter trips and the shelter medical days. The students lead games for the elementary school students and help them interact comfortably with animals. These trips, while being fun for the vet students, also expose them to community issues that they might not otherwise see. These trips also encourage the students to get involved in their own communities and give them the tools and experience that they need to do that.

4. Conclusions

The shelter program, initiated twenty years ago, started very small with an emphasis almost exclusively on spay neuter. In the twenty year history the program has grown both in size and scope. The program now includes eighteen animal shelters/humane groups and incorporates spay/neuter, basic wellness, routine diagnostics, disease management and prevention and biosecurity in the shelter environment. Furthermore, the program is teaching elementary students the value of animal life and basic health principles for animals and people.

The shelter program, while certainly benefiting the animals, the shelters, and the communities that participate, is directed towards increasing the hands-on practical skills of our veterinary graduates. Students obtain extensive experience performing surgery, performing physical examinations, conducting routine diagnostic tests, diagnosing and managing disease conditions all under direct supervision of veterinary faculty.

Acknowledgments

The authors acknowledge the individuals and organizations that have supported the development and growth of the shelter program at Mississippi State University. These include:

- Marcia Lane who endowed a Chair at the College of Veterinary Medicine to support the shelter program;
- The American Kennel Club Companion Animal Recovery (AKC_CAR) who funded, in part, the purchase and equipping of the first mobile veterinary unit;
- The Humane Society of the United States (HSUS) who provided an initial grant for operations of the program;
- PetSmart Charities, Inc. (PCI) who has provided ongoing funding for operations and funded the purchase of the second mobile veterinary unit;
- The American Society of Prevention of Cruelty to Animals (ASPVA who has provided ongoing funding for operations of the program;
- Numerous private donors who have faithfully support this program.

Author Contributions

Dr. Bushby developed the Shelter Spay Neuter Program and the Mobile Unit Program, Drs. Woodruff and Shivley developed the Shelter Medical Days and Animals in Focus Program. All three contributed to authorship of the paper.

Conflicts of Interest

The authors declare no conflict of interest.

References

1. AVMACOE Accreditation Policies and Procedures: Requirements. Available online: http://www.avma.org/ProfessionalDevelopment/Education/Accreditation/Colleges/Pages/coe-pp-requirements-of-accredited-college.aspx (accessed on 23 February 2015).
2. North American Veterinary Medical Education Consortium. Roadmap for Veterinary Medical Education in the 21st Century: Responsive, Collaborative, Flexible. Available online: http://www.aavmc.org/data/files/navmec/navmec_roadmapreport_web_single.pdf (accessed on 23 February 2015).
3. Pritchard, W.R. *Future Directions for Veterinary Medicine*; Pew National Veterinary Education Program: Durham, NC, USA, 1989; p. 189.
4. Newbury, S.; Bushby, P.A.; Cox, C.B.; Dinnage, J.D.; Griffin, B.; Hurley, K.; Isaza, N.; Jones, W.; Miller, L.; O'Quinn, J.; *et al.* Guidelines for standards of care in animal shelters. 2010. Avilable online: http://www.sheltervet.org/assets/docs/vtfasn_javma_guidelines.pdf (accessed on 23 February 2015).

5. Looney, A.L.; Bohling, M.W.; Bushby, P.A.; Howe, L.M.; Griffin, B.; Levy, J.K.; Edlestone, S.M.; Weedon, J.R.; Appel, L.D.; Rigdon-Brestle, Y.K.; *et al*. The association of shelter veterinarians veterinary medical care guidelines for spay-neuter programs. *J. Am. Vet. Med. Assoc.* **2008**, *233*, 74–86.

6. How Could You. Available online: http://cats.about.com/library/guest/ucfeature25a.htm (accessed on 23 Febraruay 2015).

7. PTS. Available online: http://www.lifewithdogs.tv/2012/04/pts/ (accessed on 23 February 2015).

8. Letter from a Shelter Manager. Available online: http://members.petfinder.com/~FL639/shelter_letter.html (accessed on 23 February 2015).

6

Hopping Down the Main Street: Eastern Grey Kangaroos at Home in an Urban Matrix

Graeme Coulson [1,2,*], **Jemma K. Cripps** [1,3] **and Michelle E. Wilson** [1,4]

[1] Department of Zoology, The University of Melbourne, Parkville, VIC 3010, Australia
[2] Macropus Consulting, 105 Canning Street, Carlton, VIC 3053, Australia
[3] Department of Environment and Primary Industries, Cnr. Midland Highway and Taylor Street, Epsom, VIC 3554, Australia; E-Mail: jemma.cripps@depi.vic.gov.au
[4] Wilson Environmental, 27 Ford Street, Brunswick, VIC 3056, Australia; E-Mail: michelle.wilson@wilsonenvironmental.com.au

* Author to whom correspondence should be addressed; E-Mails: gcoulson@unimelb.edu.au; macropusconsultingn@outlook.com.

Simple Summary: Eastern Grey Kangaroos (*Macropus giganteus*) occur throughout the seaside town of Anglesea in southern Victoria, Australia. We have tagged about half of these kangaroos in a longitudinal study of population dynamics and behavior. A golf course forms the nucleus of this population. Females live on and around the golf course, but males roam across the town in autumn and winter, living in bush reserves, empty blocks and back yards. Most females breed every year, but over half of their young disappear. Vehicles are the major cause of adult deaths, killing a much higher proportion of males than females.

Abstract: Most urban mammals are small. However, one of the largest marsupials, the Eastern Grey Kangaroo *Macropus giganteus*, occurs in some urban areas. In 2007, we embarked on a longitudinal study of this species in the seaside town of Anglesea in southern Victoria, Australia. We have captured and tagged 360 individuals to date, fitting each adult with a collar displaying its name. We have monitored survival, reproduction and movements by resighting, recapture and radio-tracking, augmented by citizen science reports of collared individuals. Kangaroos occurred throughout the town, but the golf course formed the nucleus of this urban population. The course supported a high density of kangaroos (2–5/ha), and approximately half of them were tagged. Total counts of kangaroos on the golf course were highest in summer, at the peak of the mating season, and lowest in winter, when many males but not females left the course. Almost all tagged adult females were sedentary, using only part of the golf course and adjacent native vegetation and residential blocks. In contrast, during the non-mating season (autumn and winter), many tagged adult males ranged widely across the town in a mix of native vegetation remnants, recreation reserves, vacant blocks, commercial properties and residential gardens. Annual fecundity of tagged females was generally high (≥70%), but survival of tagged juveniles was low (54%). We could not determine the cause of death of most juveniles. Vehicles were the major (47%) cause of mortality of tagged adults. Road-kills were concentrated (74%) in autumn and winter, and were heavily male biased: half of all tagged males died on roads compared with only 20% of tagged females. We predict that this novel and potent mortality factor will have profound, long-term impacts on the demography and behavior of the urban kangaroo population at Anglesea.

Keywords: Eastern Grey Kangaroo; citizen science; fecundity; habitat use; matrix-occupying; matrix sensitive; mortality; road-kill; sexual segregation; urban matrix

1. Introduction

Urbanization replaces natural environments with two novel habitat types: 'grey spaces', where >80% of the area is covered with buildings and hard surfaces, and 'green spaces', which include managed vegetation (e.g., gardens and golf courses), as well as patches of unmanaged and remnant vegetation [1]. The resulting urban matrix is characterized by different ecological processes compared with non-urban environments [2,3]. Wildlife can be classified according to their sensitivity to the grey and green components of the urban matrix: matrix-occupying, matrix-sensitive or urban-sensitive [4]. Matrix-occupying species, such as the House Mouse *Mus musculus* in England [5] and the Blackbird *Turdus merula* and Magpie *Pica pica* in Europe [6], typically dominate the urban matrix due to their ability to move through and live within the grey spaces. Matrix-sensitive species, such as the American Crow *Corvus brachyrhynchos* in the USA [7] and the European Hedgehog *Erinaceus europaeus* in England [8], perceive the grey spaces as unsuitable habitat, lacking food and shelter resources and forming a barrier to movement; these species are usually restricted to green spaces within the urban matrix, where patches of vegetation provide the only suitable habitat. The third group, urban-sensitive species such as the Small Vesper Mouse *Calomys laucha* and Azara's Grass Mouse *Akodon azarae* in Argentina [9] and the Growling Grass Frog *Litoria raniformis* in Australia [10], are unable to persist within the grey-green urban matrix, and are often threatened by urbanization.

Most research on urban wildlife has concerned birds and their use of the habitat matrix [11], but mammals have also received some attention. Baker and Harris [12] pointed out that urban mammals show a strong effect of body size on population viability: the majority of matrix-occupying and matrix-sensitive species weigh less than 10 kg, their small size allowing them to exploit a wide range of food in small habitat patches as they move easily and unobtrusively throughout the grey-green matrix. North American deer, however, are a clear exception to this pattern. White-tailed Deer *Odocoileus virginianus* have established robust populations in the urban matrix in many areas of the USA [13–17] and in Canada [18]. Its sister species, the Mule or Black-tailed Deer *Odocoileus hemionus*, has penetrated the urban matrix to a lesser extent, but has established urban populations in some areas [19,20]. The dominant management issue presented by these urban deer is the high incidence of collisions with vehicles, and their associated impacts on animal welfare, human health and property damage [16,18,21]. Furthermore, urban deer in North America often host the tick *Ixodes scapularis*, the vector of the causal agent (*Borrelia burgdorferi*) of Lyme disease [22]; the proximity of deer increases exposure to ticks, facilitating the transmission of this debilitating and sometimes fatal zoonotic disease in humans.

Macropodid marsupials (kangaroos and wallabies) are ecological analogues of deer [23], so might also be expected to occupy urban areas. Despite the common misconception that kangaroos routinely hop down the main streets of many Australian towns [24], very few urban populations have been documented. Like North American deer, the few reported cases are exceptions to the rule that most urban mammals are small (<10 kg) [12]. With females weighing ≤15 kg and males ≤21 kg [25], the Swamp Wallaby *Wallabia bicolor* occupies peri-urban patches of native vegetation around Sydney, New South Wales. [26,27]. The Agile Wallaby *Macropus agilis*, similar in size to the Swamp Wallaby [28], has also established a population in a peri-urban reserve in Darwin, Northern Territory [29]. The Western Grey Kangaroo *Macropus fuliginosus* is larger, with females weighing ≤39 kg and males ≤72 kg [30]; this species occurs on some golf courses in the suburbs of Perth, Western Australia [31]. However, all three species appear to be matrix-sensitive, since they use only the green spaces in their urban matrices. In contrast, the Eastern Grey Kangaroo *Macropus giganteus* is arguably the most urban of the macropodids, Although it is larger than the other species, with females weighing ≤42 kg and males ≤85 kg [32], it is apparently a matrix-occupying species in some parts of its range, using both grey and green spaces within the matrix. The best-known population of Eastern Grey Kangaroos lives within and on the fringe of the city of Canberra, Australian Capital Territory, which is known as 'the bush capital' [33]. Ballard [34] also described a population living amongst a retirement community in Port Macquarie on the north coast of New South Wales, and Inwood *et al.* [35] reported another urban population in Anglesea on the west coast of Victoria. Social surveys at these three sites revealed that collisions with vehicles were the dominant management issue, as for North American deer, but people were also concerned about the risk of attacks by kangaroos [33–35].

The urban kangaroo population at Anglesea is the subject of a community-based management program, developed in response to the issues raised by the human residents [35]. Three key issues that emerged were: (1) improved understanding of the biology of Anglesea's kangaroos, particularly their health, demographics and movements; (2) monitoring biological change over time, and assessing the outcomes of management actions; (3) mitigation of kangaroo-vehicle collisions by identifying hotspots. In 2007 we began a program of applied research aimed at addressing these issues. We adopted a longitudinal approach, capturing and marking a large sample of the population [36], then monitoring these individuals through time. Studies such as these have proven valuable in a variety of wildlife species [37], but a long-term project on marked kangaroos had not previously been undertaken. Crucially for our project, we named each individual and displayed its name on its collar, then used conventional monitoring techniques augmented by citizen science reports to monitor individuals [38]. This marked population formed the foundation for ancillary studies of the efficacy of anthelmintic drugs [39] and contraceptive implants [40], and the effect of reproduction on feeding behavior [41], which have contributed to the overall research program. We have also coupled the Anglesea program with a second longitudinal study, commenced in 2008, of a more natural population at Wilsons Promontory National Park, southern Victoria. Projects are underway at both sites on factors influencing the age at maturity, timing of births, sex ratio of young, and reproductive success of both sexes. This paper reports on our first six years of urban kangaroo research at Anglesea, and assesses our progress towards the three key issues of concern to Anglesea residents.

2. Methods

Anglesea (38°40'S, 144°19'E) is located on the Surf Coast in southern Victoria, Australia (Figure 1). The town has about 2000 permanent human residents; the population increases at weekends and rises dramatically during summer, exceeding 10,000 at peak times [42]. Anglesea lies on the iconic Great Ocean Road, a major attraction for domestic and international tourists, and many include kangaroo viewing in their itinerary. Kangaroo imagery promotes the town: banners in the main street declare Anglesea to be 'where bush meets sea', the Anglesea Primary School boasts a 'kangaroo on a surfboard' logo, and the Anglesea Golf Club features a kangaroo on its flag and signage around the course. The town has a riverside park as well as a number of small reserves of remnant native vegetation within the urban matrix. The Surf Coast Shire, the local government authority, imposes strict regulations against clearing of vegetation on private land, and many residential blocks are well vegetated. Many blocks are unfenced and some streets are unsealed. The urban area lies within the Anglesea Heath; this forms part of the Great Otway National Park, which is an extensive, continuous reserve of native vegetation along much of the Great Ocean Road. Anglesea Heath is jointly managed by Parks Victoria and Alcoa Australia, which operates an open-cast brown coal mine and coal-fired power station in the heath north of the town [43].

2.1. Study Sites

The Anglesea Golf Club has an 18-hole course of tree-lined fairways (Figure 2) planted with Couch Grass *Cynodon dactylon*, which is irrigated and fertilized, as are the tees and greens. The Front Nine (holes 1–9) is 32 ha in area, including practice areas and a Couch Grass nursery. The Front Nine is bounded to the north and west by the Anglesea Heath, an extensive area of native vegetation dominated by eucalypts with an understory of low shrubs. Its southern side is bounded partly by a band of remnant native woodland bordering residential streets, and by the entrance road to the clubhouse; the eastern side is bounded by Golf Links Road, with houses on the opposite side. The Front Nine is unfenced, so kangaroos can move freely in all directions across these boundaries. The Back Nine (holes 10–18) is 27 ha in area. It is bounded to the south and west by houses facing away from the course; many are unfenced so kangaroos can move through the yards onto residential streets. Its northern and western sides are demarcated by a 1.8-m high steel mesh fence, which is designed to stop kangaroos moving onto Golf Links Road and the entrance road, and to restrict access to the course by tourists. Each half of the course has a 2-ha patch of remnant native vegetation, roughly in the center, providing additional refuge for the kangaroos.

Camp Wilkin is a 6-ha school camp at the junction of Golf Links Road and Noble Street, located on the opposite side of the fence road bordering the Back Nine of the golf course. The camp consists of a building complex (bunkrooms, dining room, gymnasium, and staff housing) at the corner of two residential streets, as well as a sports field, adventure equipment and remnant native vegetation at the rear of the camp, where kangaroos shelter during the day. The perimeter of the camp has a tall paling fence on two sides, which effectively contains kangaroos, and a low wire fence on the other two sides, which they can hop over. However, most kangaroo movement occurs onto the streets through vehicle gates.

Figure 1. Aerial photograph of Anglesea, Victoria, Australia, showing the compact residential area bounded by the Anglesea Heath, the Anglesea Golf Club (Golf) within the town boundary, and the Alcoa Australia coal mine and power station (Alcoa) to the north of the town. Also shows locations of road-kills of tagged male and female Eastern Grey Kangaroos *Macropus giganteus* reported from 2008 to 2013.

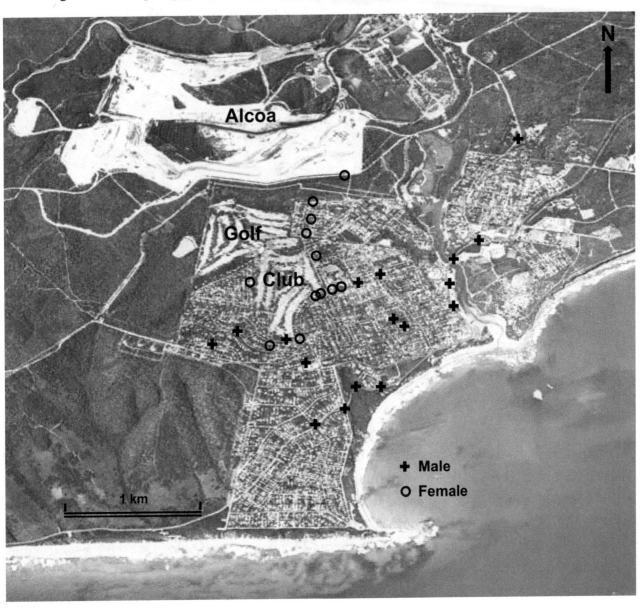

Figure 2. Aerial photograph of the Anglesea Golf Club, Victoria, Australia, showing the layout of the 18-hole course and the contrast between open foraging areas and vegetated shelter for Eastern Grey Kangaroos *Macropus giganteus*.

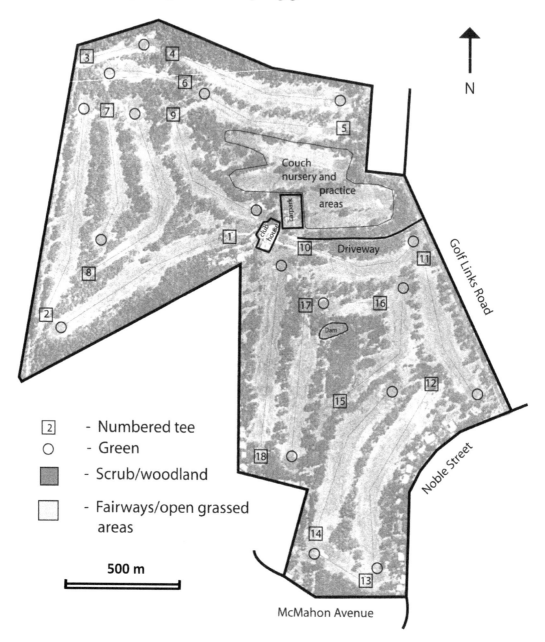

2.2. Capture and Marking

To capture kangaroos we exploited their habituation to people on the golf course and at the school camp, using two techniques that have proven to be safe and selective. For captures at close range we used a 10-mL Paxarms syringe attached to a light-weight telescopic pole [36]. The smallest of these was a two-piece aluminum pole, which extended to 1.4 m and superficially resembled a golf club. For less approachable individuals we used longer (≤3.6 m) two-piece poles, or even longer (≤5.3 m) three-piece poles if necessary. We approached kangaroos slowly and injected Zoletil 100 (1:1 Zolezapam and Tiletamine) into the muscle mass of the hind-limb at a dose rate of approximately 5 mg/kg. Adult kangaroos that were newly arrived at the golf course were often too wary to capture with a pole syringe, as were some individuals that had been captured repeatedly. We captured these individuals using a WildVet Para-medic band-powered bow (range ≤ 8 m) or a WildVet Pro-medic crossbow (range ≤ 20 m). Both bows fired lightweight injection arrows into the hind-limb muscle with minimum impact trauma, and injected a dose of approximately 5 mg/kg of Zoletil 100.

To date we have captured and marked 360 individual kangaroos: 211 (68 male, 143 female) as adults, 15 (8 male, 7 female) as sub-adults, and 39 as young-at-foot (22 male, 17 female) closely associated with their mothers after pouch exit. In addition, 83 young in the pouch (55 male, 37 female) were large enough to tag when we captured their mothers. We have recaptured adults on 269 occasions, comprising one (57% of adult recaptures), two (28%), three (10%), four (4%) or five (1%) recaptures per individual. We have also recaptured 40 sub-adults up to three times each, and 39 young-at-foot once or twice each. All but 17 of our captures of adults, sub-adults and young-at-foot were on the golf course; we captured most (16) of the others at Camp Wilkin, plus one in a small reserve beside the Anglesea River. We used the small pole for the majority (56%) of captures, two medium poles for 20% of captures and two long poles for 19% of captures. For the remainder of captures of more wary kangaroos we used either the Para-medic bow (4%) of the more powerful Pro-medic bow (2%).

Once a kangaroo had been injected by pole syringe or arrow, we withdrew a short distance and kept the kangaroo under observation to guard against approaches by people, dogs, cars or aggressive conspecifics, and intervened when necessary on occasions. Induction was rapid (about 5 min), resulting in immobilisation and anaesthesia for approximately 1 h. When the kangaroo was immobilised, we transferred it to a shade-cloth cradle to weigh it, and took a standard set of body measurements. We marked each adult and sub-adult with a unique combination of two or three colored Allflex ear-tags, with an individual identity number and enhanced by color-matched 3M reflective tape for identification at night. If pouch young were furred and had erect ears, we marked them with a unique color combination of two Leader swivel tags, which we also numbered and matched with reflective tape. We followed the same procedure for a few young-at-foot, which we captured soon after they had left the pouch permanently. Insertion of the Allflex and Leader tags displaced a small piece of ear tissue, which we collected for genetic analysis. We fitted each adult male with a 45-mm wide collar made of Ritchey trilaminar plastic, overlapped and fastened with two steel nuts and bolts; this design proved moderately resistant to damage incurred during fights between males. We fitted some adult females with 35-mm wide collars of this material, but gave most a softer and more flexible 35-mm wide collar made of a doubled strip of Innova International UV-stable vinyl, overlapped and fastened with four pairs of ITW Fastex ratchet rivets. We gave each individual a unique three, four or sometimes five-letter name (e.g., *Nat* and *Vlad*), and wrote the name in large letters with a black Allflex tag pen two or three times around the collar. After examination and marking, we moved each kangaroo to a quiet, sheltered area and allowed it to recover without further disturbance.

2.3. Population Surveys

In 2010 we began twice-yearly surveys of the golf course population, one in winter and another in late summer. Two of us (GC and JC) conducted total counts of kangaroos in the morning, starting at the beginning of civil twilight, and in the evening, starting 1.5 h before the end of civil twilight, when most kangaroos were feeding in the open on the fairways. We modified the procedure used by

Inwood *et al.* [33]: instead of walking along all the fairways in the order of play, we walked steadily along the trees lining the fairways so that we could effectively scan pairs of fairways, thus minimizing potential double-counting of kangaroos that moved between fairways and allowing us to cover the course more rapidly at the optimal time of day. We used binoculars to scan groups of kangaroos from distances ≤50 m, counting all adults, sub-adults and young-at-foot, but excluding young that temporarily emerged from the pouch. From the start of 2011 we also recorded each individual as marked (with ear-tags and/or collar) or not. To have two independent counts for each side, we each started on opposite sides of the course, then swapped to the alternate side. We discounted any surveys where an obvious disturbance (e.g., by grounds staff or dogs) might have caused a double count. We took the higher of our two counts on each side as the total for each morning or evening session, and took the highest session total as the minimum population size for each survey period.

At least once each season we conducted a census of the kangaroo population at the Golf Club and at Camp Wilkin, augmented by occasional sightings away from these focal areas (see Section 2.4. Movements). We recorded the presence of each marked individual and its location on the golf course or school camp. We also recorded the reproductive status of each female, any loss of tags or collars, and any obvious injuries or marked changes in body condition or behavior.

2.4. Movements

We obtained data on the movements of marked kangaroos beyond the golf course from five sources: citizen science reports, street searches, camera traps, road-kills and radio-tracking. Naming the kangaroos and displaying the names on their collars proved to be a key element in engaging public interest in our research program [38]. To encourage citizen science reports of marked kangaroos around the town, we gave talks to a range of community groups and to all year levels at the local primary school, and spoke about the program at other events during the year. We also put up posters in shop windows and community noticeboards, and distributed contact cards to local organizations and interested individuals. In addition, our research program was covered by television documentaries, local newspapers and community newsletters.

We conducted searches of the streets around the town from a vehicle, aided by a spotlight at night. With experience, we were able to identify a number of locations where kangaroos could usually be seen, and returned to them often. Road-kills of marked kangaroos were reported by members of the public, wildlife carers and local police, who were often called out to shoot badly-injured kangaroos [35].

In the autumn of 2012 we selected five marked adult males that were often not present on the golf course, with the goal of qualitatively assessing the types of habitats occupied. We recaptured them and fitted them with a reflective Sirtrack radio-collar. The collars weighed <250 g, incorporated a mortality switch, and transmitted in the 150–151 MHz band with a range of approximately 1.5 km. In the following winter we tracked them at irregular intervals at night and during the day. We located each individual off the golf course two to seven times, initially by triangulation from vantage points or by driving around the town with an omnidirectional antenna on the roof of the vehicle, then by homing in on foot. Once we had located them, we recorded the habitat they occupied and the identity of any other marked kangaroos nearby.

2.5. Mortality

We found some carcasses of marked kangaroos on the golf course and nearby streets. However, most deaths of marked kangaroos were reported to us by Golf Club staff, police, wildlife carers and concerned residents. When a carcass was found, we confirmed the kangaroo's identity from its ear-tags and/or collar, recorded its location, and determined its cause of death when possible. We also attempted to retrieve its body and take the same morphometric measures recorded in life, except where the body parts were damaged, then removed the head and allowed it to decompose so that we could later age the clean skull by molar index [44]. In three cases when the carcass was fresh and the cause of death was unclear, we submitted the kangaroo for formal post-mortem examination.

3. Results

3.1. Abundance and Attendance

The abundance of kangaroos on the golf course declined by about 100 animals in the last decade, from a peak of 359 in summer 2004 to 237–263 in the last four summers (Figure 3). Winter counts have shown a similar decline, from 290 in 2006 to 142–210 in the last four winters (Figure 3). An oscillating pattern of winter troughs and summer peaks in abundance has also been evident since twice-yearly surveys began in 2010. In the last seven surveys, 46–66% of the kangaroos seen were tagged (Figure 3).

Figure 3. Abundance of Eastern Grey Kangaroos *Macropus giganteus* at Anglesea Golf Club from surveys conducted in winter and summer, inconsistently at first, from 2004 to 2014. Data for 2004 and 2006 compiled from Inwood *et al.* [35].

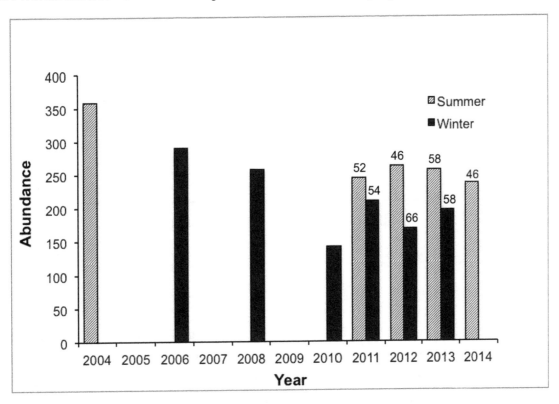

To assess the attendance of tagged kangaroos at the golf course, we scored individuals as present or absent in each census from May 2008 to November 2013. We included only censuses that recorded ≥50 tagged adults to ensure an adequate sample size. This gave eight censuses in autumn and winter (March to August), two in each year of the four years, and 16 censuses in spring and summer (September to February), spread almost evenly over the years. We scored only individuals tagged as adults (76 females and 34 males), from the first census after each individual was tagged to the last census in which it was known to be alive, excluding individuals that spanned <10 censuses to ensure adequate coverage of the two 'seasons'. The overall attendance rate was high, with a mean (±SE) of $79 \pm 1\%$ (Figure 4). Attendance was not affected by season (Repeated-measures ANOVA, F = 0.51, df = 1,108, P = 0.478), but the attendance rate of females was higher than males (F = 25.25 df = 1,108, P < 0.0001). Season and sex also interacted (F = 15.48, df = 1,108, P = 0.0001): attendance by males was much lower in autumn-winter (62%) than in spring-summer (75%), whereas females remained above 80%.

Figure 4. Mean attendance rate of individual male and female Eastern Grey Kangaroos *Macropus giganteus* (tagged as adults) in autumn/winter and spring/summer on the Anglesea golf course from May 2008 to November 2013. Data from censuses recording ≥50 tagged adults (8 autumn/winter and 16 spring/summer), from the first census after each individual was tagged to the last in which it was known to be alive, excluding individuals spanning <10 censuses. Error bars show standard error.

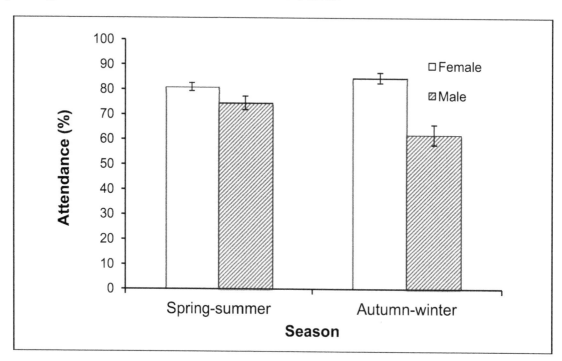

3.2. Fecundity and Mortality

We recorded the number of reproductive attempts by each tagged female based mainly on a visible bulge indicative of a young in the pouch. In some cases, pouch young were too small to detect externally but were recorded when we captured the female. The overall level of fecundity of adult females was low in the first two full years of this study: 39% in 2008 (n = 77) and 38% in 2009 (n = 65). Fecundity in the following four years was consistently higher: 70% in 2010 (n = 96), 76% in 2011 (n = 91), 74% in 2012 (n = 78) and 75% in 2013 (n = 63). These values excluded any of the females treated with fertility control implants by Wilson et al. [40], but included females used as procedural (untreated) controls in that study.

A high proportion (46%) of the 221 juveniles that we tagged subsequently disappeared from the population before the age of three years. Although we rarely found their carcasses, we concluded that these juveniles had died, because they were still dependent on, or closely associated with, their mothers at the time. Of these juveniles, 41% disappeared in their first year, mostly towards the end of the ten-month pouch life, 54% in their second year, and the remainder (4%) in their third year.

Adult mortality could not be distinguished from dispersal from the golf course or school camp, so we did not estimate the mortality rate of adults. However, we were able to confirm the deaths of 78 tagged adults. More than half (55%) of these were found dead on the golf course, or on streets or in reserves elsewhere in the town. The other cases involved seriously injured or moribund kangaroos on the golf course or around the town, which were either shot by police (31%) or given lethal injections by wildlife rescuers (14%). The sex ratio (1 male:1.53 females) of recorded deaths did not differ from the ratio of adults originally tagged (Contingency Chi square, χ^2 = 2.86, df = 1, P = 0.091. The estimated age of the skulls of adults that we retrieved (n = 23) ranged from 2.8 to 18.7 (median = 8.9) years. We were unable to determine the direct cause of 53% of adult deaths. One died when struck by a golf ball, five sustained traumatic injuries from unknown sources, and four were probably attacked by Dogs or European Foxes Vulpes vulpes, which were present on the golf course at the time.

Collisions with vehicles were the major (47%) known cause of death. These road-kills had a strong seasonal bias: of 37 incidents that could be assigned to a season, 32% occurred in autumn and 41% in winter, whereas only 14% occurred in each of spring and summer (Goodness-of-fit G-test, G = 42.85, df = 3, P < 0.0001). However, there was no difference in the frequency on weekdays versus weekends for the 29 incidents assigned to a specific day (Goodness-of-fit G-test, G = 0.29, df = 1, P = 0.594). Unlike overall deaths, collisions were highly sex biased: exactly half of all males originally tagged as adult died on roads, versus 20% of adult females tagged (Contingency Chi-square, χ^2 = 20.55, df = 1, P < 0.0001). The spatial distribution of road-kills also differed markedly between the sexes: with the exception of one female (Grace) on the edge of town and 0.5 km from the golf course, all road-kills of females were on streets within a block of the golf course, whereas males were killed throughout the town (Figure 1).

3.3. Movement and Habitats

Tagged kangaroos moved between the golf course and Camp Wilkin. Of the ten individuals first captured at Camp Wilkin, we resighted five (all female) only at the camp, but saw the others (three male, two female) on the golf course on occasions. Another seven individuals (four male, two female) that had first been captured on the golf course were seen at Camp Wilkin. We also received citizen science reports of tagged kangaroos, primarily males, throughout the town, and augmented these with our own observations (Figure 5). In addition, we located radio-collared males in many parts of the town, and radio-tracking one individual often led us to other tagged males nearby. These movements off the golf course and into the town matrix occurred mainly in autumn and winter. Males sometimes also left the golf course in summer. For example, one large male (*Stan*) was reported resting during the day and drinking from a pond in a shady backyard on hot (>40 °C) days in two consecutive summers. However, we had insufficient locations of tagged individuals for quantitative analyses of habitat use. At a qualitative level, kangaroos occurred in a wide range of habitats beyond the golf course and school camp: bush reserves, public playgrounds, holiday parks, vacant blocks, commercial properties and residential gardens. We also located some kangaroos in native vegetation of the Anglesea Heath on the fringe of the town.

Figure 5. Two tagged and collared male Eastern Grey Kangaroos *Macropus giganteus* (*Otis* and *Pete*) at the Anglesea Lookout Flora Reserve above the Great Ocean Road, about 1 km south of where they were collared and tagged at the Anglesea Golf Club.

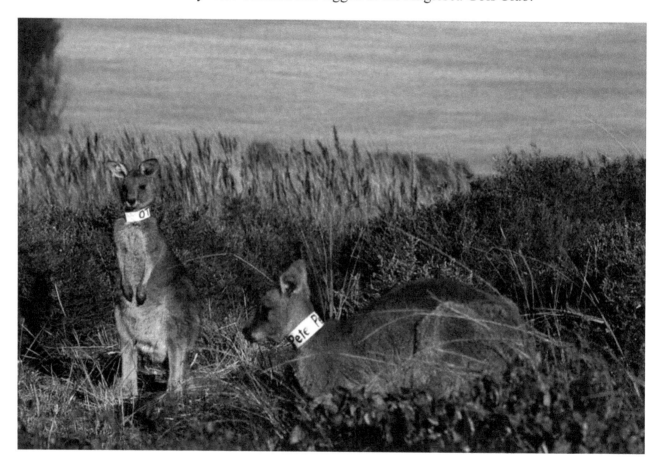

We detected only four tagged kangaroos moving beyond the town boundary. One young adult male (*Max*) was killed by a car on the Great Ocean Road, 3.4 km northeast of his last sighting on the golf course. A second male (*Ben*) was reported a number of times in the neighboring town of Aireys Inlet, 6.6 km southwest of the golf course, and was ultimately found dead 12 months after initial reports, on the Great Ocean Road on the edge of Aireys Inlet. One young female (*Boo*) was detected on a camera trap set for a fauna survey in the Anglesea Heath, 8.6 km north-northwest of the golf course and three years after we last saw her there. A second adult female (*Vahn*) was detected on another camera trap set to monitor European Foxes in the Anglesea Heath, 7.7 km west of the golf course, and 4 months after her last sighting on the course.

4. Discussion

Many wildlife species exhibit adaptations to the novel and often-stressful conditions they experience in urban environments [6,45]. For example, long-term studies of Florida Key Deer *Odocoileus virginianus clavium* show that they have adapted to urbanization by increasing their use of urban habitat, and their body weight and survival is now higher than in less urban deer [15]. However, long-term studies of urban wildlife are extremely rare in Australia [4]. As the first long-term study of tagged Eastern Grey Kangaroos, our set of findings cannot yet be contrasted with the demography and behavior of other kangaroo populations in more natural settings. Our study also has many years to run, and we cannot yet determine the extent of demographic or behavioral change within the kangaroo population at Anglesea. Nonetheless, we can explore some elements of kangaroo ecology at Anglesea and identify potential effects of urbanization.

4.1. Population Dynamics

The density of the kangaroo population on the 73-ha golf course has ranged from 4.9/ha at its peak in summer 2003–04 to 2.0/ha in winter 2010, when we began twice-yearly surveys. The density in summer has since ranged from 3.3/ha to 3.6/ha. These densities were equal to or higher than any in the peri-urban reserves reviewed by Adderton Herbert [46], and are similar to the maximum densities recorded in the Australian Capital Territory [33]. These comparisons suggest that the population density of kangaroos can be enhanced by the urban environment, as it has been for many wildlife species elsewhere in the world [6,15].

The decline in abundance since the peak in summer 2003–04 has no obvious cause. A sample of 42 adult female kangaroos was treated with contraceptive implants in 2008 as part of an ancillary study of fertility control techniques [40,41]. The efficacy of one compound (deslorelin) was limited to one or two years, whereas the other (levonorgestrel) has continued to be effective [47]. However, this experiment also included 23 control (untreated) females, and other females, both tagged and untagged, were not treated with contraceptives. It is unlikely that fertility control caused the population to decline, because to achieve population stability in a long-lived, annually-breeding species like the Eastern Grey Kangaroo, it is necessary to contracept a high proportion (>90%) of a population [48]. A more likely explanation for the decline is that the kangaroo population at Anglesea was under pressure from the 'millennium drought', a long-term rainfall deficit across south-eastern Australia from 2001 to 2009 [49]. While the permanent water and irrigated fairways on the golf course would have buffered the kangaroo population against drought, the course may not have been able to support densities approaching 5/ha indefinitely. Anecdotal observations of kangaroos feeding on roadside verges, and an increase in fatal incidents reported by police over a decade [35], support this interpretation. The unusually low fecundity (<40%) of adult females in 2008 and 2009 was also consistent with the impact of drought in other populations of Eastern Grey Kangaroos [50].

A pattern of summer peaks and winter troughs in abundance has been evident since 2010. Breeding is seasonal at Anglesea [40], with a peak of births in early summer generating a pulse in recruitment as young leave the pouch permanently the following spring. However, young tagged in the pouch disappeared at a high rate (46%), and 41% of those were in their first year, so any recruitment pulse would likely have been muted by the time we conducted population surveys later in summer. Banks [51] reported a similar rate of loss of juvenile Eastern Grey Kangaroos, which he attributed to predation by European foxes. The subsequent trough in winter would reflect a combination of continued disappearance (54%) of juveniles in their second year, coupled with the lower attendance rate (61%) of adult males on the golf course.

4.2. Movement

We detected very few large-scale movements of tagged kangaroos. However, our reliance on citizen science reports, augmented by our own sightings, undoubtedly generated a detectability bias. While the dispersal and subsequent road-kills of two young males (*Max* and *Ben*) were reported by citizen scientists, the long-range movements into the Anglesea Heath by two adult females (*Boo* and *Vahn*) would have gone undetected without camera traps set for other purposes. However, other movement studies of Eastern Grey Kangaroos, based either on sightings of tagged individuals [52] or radio-tracking [53–55], have also shown that they are largely sedentary. We are unable to assess whether the home range size of kangaroos in the urban matrix of Anglesea is smaller than in more natural landscapes, as has been reported for well-studied white-tailed deer [15,56,57].

Adult males exhibited strong sexual segregation in space, as reported for this species in natural landscapes [58]. The attendance of females on the golf course was high throughout the year, whereas attendance of males declined in the non-breeding season (autumn and winter). Males were then more likely to be encountered throughout the town in a variety of habitats, and road-kills of males were widespread across the town, unlike those of females, which were almost all near the golf course. The incidence of road-kills was considerably higher in the non-breeding season, when 73% of deaths occurred. The incidence of road-kills was also heavily biased towards males. Similar male bias in the frequency of road-kills has been reported for Eastern Grey Kangaroos in the peri-urban landscape around Canberra [59] and in rural landscapes [60,61]. However, these studies lacked data on the sex composition of the populations from which the road-kills were drawn, so could not assess the impact of vehicles as a sex-biased mortality factor. At Anglesea, the impact was clearly male biased: half of the males that we tagged were definitely killed on roads, whereas only one fifth of tagged females were.

5. Conclusions

The Eastern Grey Kangaroo has a broad geographic distribution, and occurs in a wide variety of habitats, ranging from native forests, woodlands (including mallee scrub), shrublands and heathland, to modified habitats such as pine plantations and golf courses [32]. These habitats all provide a mix open grassy foraging areas and cover from the weather and predators [32]. At a landscape scale, the density of this species is highest when these dual resources occur in a mosaic, so that forage and cover are in close proximity [62]. Our study at Anglesea suggests that the urban matrix also provides a suitable mosaic of forage and cover, and that kangaroos are able to move through and live within the matrix at the scale of a residential block. Therefore the kangaroos of Anglesea can be classified as matrix-occupying [4] and, like North American deer, do not conform to predictions based on body size [15]. However, our study shows that the golf course forms the nucleus of this population.

The nearby school camp (Camp Wilkin) supports a satellite sub-population, exchanging individuals with the golf course, but we are confident that there is no other source of kangaroos anywhere in the town.

Although Eastern Grey Kangaroos occupied the urban matrix in Anglesea, strong sex differences were evident. Females exploited the mix of forage and cover provided by the golf course and adjacent residential blocks; males were less reliant on the golf course and moved further away during autumn and winter, occupying small patches of forage and cover throughout the town. This disparity suggests that, like urban Coyotes *Canis latrans* in North America [63], kangaroos have retained their mating system in this urban matrix. Kangaroos are polygynous and show sexual segregation during the non-mating season [58]. In this urban environment, the segregative behavior of males exposes them to greater risk of road-kill, and probably to other disturbance from people and Dogs. This novel and potent mortality factor, which operates selectively against males, is likely to have profound impacts on the demography and behavioral ecology of urban kangaroos in the future.

The aim of this study was to address the three key kangaroo issues raised by the human residents of Anglesea. The first of these issues was a desire to understand more of the biology of Anglesea's kangaroos, particularly their health, demographics and movements. Animal health remains poorly understood, although an ancillary study [64] has examined the influence of gastrointestinal parasites on growth, body condition and haematological values of juvenile kangaroos at Anglesea. We now have a more complete understanding of the demography of this population, notably the generally high rate of female fecundity, which is largely offset by high juvenile mortality. Nevertheless, we have been unable to elucidate the causes of mortality in roughly half of adults and juveniles. Our sightings and citizen science reports of tagged kangaroos have revealed strong sex differences in ranging behavior, and radio-tracking a small sample of adult males has further illuminated their use of the urban matrix. However, we frequently encountered logistical challenges posed by radio interference and trespass onto private property, which are typical of radio-tracking in urban environments [65,66], so we have begun a pilot study of Global Positioning System collars (fitted to one male and one female), designed to log locations at 30-min intervals for 18 months. The second issue was the need to monitor biological change over time, and assess the outcomes of management actions. Our twice-yearly surveys of the kangaroo population on the golf course have shown a long-term decline in abundance, although its underlying causes are obscure, and strong seasonal oscillation in use of the course by adult males. No specific management actions have been undertaken since we began this study, but we now have a solid information base to assess management outcomes. The final management issue was mitigation of kangaroo-vehicle collisions by identifying hotspots. Road-kills have proven to be a dominant mortality factor, and several hotspots can now be identified. More importantly, our finding of strong spatial segregation by adult males in the autumn and winter non-breeding season has clear implications for the human residents: collisions with large male kangaroos can occur throughout the town on any day in half of the year. This point will become a key message in learning to live with kangaroos in Anglesea.

Acknowledgments

We are grateful to Helen Catanchin and Danielle Inwood, whose work with the community laid the foundations for this study, and to Teigan Allen, who helped to launch the capture program. A number of people have since captured kangaroos (Clare Death, Marco Festa-Bianchet, Sarah Garnick, Uriel

Gélin, Camille Le Gall-Payne and Allison McKay) with us, and many others have assisted with animal handling. The Anglesea and Aireys Inlet Kangaroo Advisory Group encouraged this project from the outset and kept a watchful eye on it. The managers of Anglesea Golf Club, Damian Franzmann and Rachel Kane, have been supportive throughout the project. The YMCA, Camp Wilkin, and Heather and David Oke have generously provided accommodation. Marco Festa-Bianchet made valuable comments on the manuscript. Elements of this study were funded by the Department of Sustainability and Environment, Holsworth Wildlife Research Endowment, Parks Victoria's Research Partners Panel, and Koala and Kangaroo Contraception Program (ARC Linkage Project 0560344) led by the late Prof Des Cooper. Animal capture and handling was approved by The University of Melbourne Animal Ethics Committee (Ethics ID 06146, 0703882, 1011709) and the Department of Sustainability and Environment (research permits 10004041, 10004256, 10005557).

Author Contributions

Graeme Coulson supervised the research program and wrote most of the text. Most of the fieldwork was conducted by Graeme Coulson in 2007, Michelle Wilson in 2008–2009 and Jemma Cripps in 2010–2013.

Conflicts of Interest

The authors declare no conflict of interest.

References and Notes

1. Adams, C.E.; Lindsey, K.J.; Ash, S.J. *Urban Wildlife Management*; Taylor & Francis: Boca Raton, FL, USA, 2006.

2. McDonnell, M.J.; Pickett, S.T. A. Ecosystem structure and function along urban-rural gradients: An unexploited opportunity for ecology. *Ecology* **1990**, *71*, 1232–1327.

3. Collins, J.P.; Kinzing, A.; Grimm, N.B.; Fagan, W.F.; Hope, D.; Wu, J.; Borer, E.T. A new urban ecology. *Am. Sci.* **2000**, *88*, 416–426.

4. Garden, J.; McAlpine, C.; Peterson, A.; Jones, D.; Possingham, H. Review of the ecology of Australian urban fauna: A focus on spatially explicit processes. *Aust. Ecol.* **2006**, *31*, 126–148.

5. Berry, R.J. Town Mouse, Country Mouse: adaptation and adaptability in *Mus domesticus (M. musculus domesticus)*. *Mamm. Rev.* **1981**, *11*, 91–136.

6. Luniak, M. Synurbization—Adaptation of animal wildlife to urban development. In *Proceedings of the 4th International Symposium on Urban Wildlife Conservation*; Shaw, W.W., Harris, L.K., VanDruff, L., Eds.; University of Arizona: Tucson, AZ, USA, 2004; pp. 267–269.

7. Withey, J.C.; Marzluff, J.W. Multi-scale use of lands providing anthropogenic resources by American Crows in an urbanizing landscape. *Landscape Ecol.* **2009**, *24*, 281–293

8. Dowding, C.V.; Harris, S.; Poulton, S.; Baker, P.J. Nocturnal ranging behavior of urban hedgehogs, *Erinaceus europaeus*, in relation to risk and reward. *Anim. Behav.* **2010**, *80*, 13–21.

9. Cavia, R.; Cueto, G.R.; Olga Virginia Suárez, O.V. Changes in rodent communities according to the landscape structure in an urban ecosystem. *Landscape Urban Plan.* **2009**, *90*, 11–19.

10. Heard, G.W.; McCarthy, M.A.; Scroggie, M.P.; Baumgartner, J.B.; Parris, K.M. A Bayesian model of metapopulation viability, with application to an endangered amphibian. *Divers. Distrib.* **2013**, *19*, 555–566.

11. Adams, L.W. Urban wildlife ecology and conservation: A brief history of the discipline. *Urban Ecosyst.* **2005**, *8*, 139–156.

12. Baker, P.J.; Harris, S. Urban mammals: What does the future hold? An analysis of the factors affecting patterns of use of residential gardens in Great Britain. *Mammal Rev.* **2007**, *37*, 297–315.

13. Etter, D.R.; Hollis, K.M.; Van Deelen, T.R.; Ludwig, D.R.; Chelsvig, J.E.; Anchor, C.L.; Warner, R.E. Survival and movements of white-tailed deer in suburban Chicago, Illinois. *J. Wildl. Manage.* **2002**, *66*, 500–510.

14. Porter, W.F.; Underwood, B.; Woodard, J.L. Movement behavior, dispersal, and the potential for localized management of deer in a suburban environment. *J. Wildl. Manage.* **2004**, *68*, 247–256.

15. Harveson, P.M.; Lopez, R.R.; Collier, B.A.; Silvy, N.J. Impacts of urbanization on Florida Key deer behavior and population dynamics. *Biol. Cons.* **2007**, *134*, 321–331.

16. DeNicola, A.J.; Williams, S.C. Sharpshooting suburban white-tailed deer reduces deer–vehicle collisions. *Human-Wildl. Confl.* **2008**, *2*, 28–33.

17. Walter, W.D.; Beringer, J.; Hansen, L.P.; Fischer, J.W.; Millspaugh, J.P.; Vercauteren, K.C. Factors affecting space use overlap by white-tailed deer in an urban landscape. *Int. J. Geogr. Inf. Sci.* **2011**, *25*, 379–392.

18. Ng, J.W.; Nielsen, C.; St.Clair, C.C. Landscape and traffic factors influencing deer–vehicle collisions in an urban environment. *Human-Wildl. Confl.* **2008**, *2*, 34–47.

19. McCullough, D.R.; Jennings, K.W.; Gates, N.B.; Elliott, B.G.; DiDonato, J.E. Overabundant deer populations in California. *Wildl. Soc. Bull.* **1997**, *25*, 478–483.

20. Wolfe, L.L.; Miller, M.W.; Williams, E.S. Feasibility of "test-and-cull" for managing chronic wasting disease in urban mule deer. *Wildl. Soc. Bull.* **2004**, *32*, 500–505.

21. Nielsen, C.K.; Anderson, R.G.; Grund, M.D. Landscape influences on deer-vehicle accident areas in an urban environment. *J. Wildl. Manage.* **2003**, *67*, 46–51.

22. Magnarelli, L.A.; Denicola, A.; Stafford; K.C.; Anderson, J.F., III. *Borrelia burgdorferi* in an urban environment: White-tailed deer with infected ticks and antibodies. *J. Clin. Microbiol.* **1995**, *33*, 541–544.

23. Jarman, P.J. Social behavior and organization in the Macropodoidea. *Adv. Stud. Behav.* **1991**, *20*, 1–50.

24. Exley, B. Kangaroos on the main street? Using resources to break down stereotypes. *Jigsaw: Mag. Fam. Day Care Aust.* **2005**, *35*, 9–10.

25. Merchant, J.C. Swamp wallaby *Wallabia bicolor*. In *The Mammals of Australia*, 3rd ed.; Van Dyck, S., Strahan, R., Eds.; Reed New Holland: Sydney, Australia, 2008; pp. 323–324.

26. Ramp, D.; Ben-Ami, D. The effect of road-based fatalities on the viability of a peri-urban swamp wallaby population. *J. Wildl. Manage.* **2006**, *70*, 1615–1624.

27. Garvey, N.; Ben-Ami, D.; Ramp, D.; Croft, D B. Survival behavior of swamp wallabies during prescribed burning and wildfire. *Wildl. Res.* **2010**, *37*, 1–12.

28. Merchant, J.C. Agile wallaby *Macropus agilis*. In *The Mammals of Australia*, 3rd ed.; Van Dyck, S., Strahan, R., Eds.; Reed New Holland: Sydney, Australia, 2008; pp. 404–406.

29. Stirrat, S.C. Seasonal changes in home-range area and habitat use by the agile wallaby (*Macropus agilis*). *Wildl. Res.* **2003**, *30*, 593–600.

30. Coulson, G. Western grey kangaroo *Macropus fuliginosus*. In *The Mammals of Australia*, 3rd ed.; Van Dyck, S., Strahan, R., Eds.; Reed New Holland: Sydney, Australia, 2008; pp. 333–334.

31. Mayberry, C.; Maloney, S.K.; Mitchell, J.; Mawson, P.; Bencini, R. Reproductive implications of exposure to *Toxoplasma gondii* and *Neospora caninum* in western grey kangaroos (*Macropus fuliginosus ocydromus*). *J. Wildl. Dis.* **2014**, *50*, 364–368.

32. Coulson, G. Eastern grey kangaroo *Macropus giganteus*. In *The Mammals of Australia*, 3rd ed.; Van Dyck, S., Strahan, R., Eds.; Reed New Holland: Sydney, Australia, 2008; pp. 335–338.

33. Australian Capital Territory. *ACT Kangaroo Management Plan*; Territory and Municipal Services: Canberra, Australia, 2010.

34. Ballard, G. Peri-urban kangaroos. Wanted? Dead or alive? In *Too Close for Comfort: Contentious Issues in Human-Wildlife Encounters*; Lunney, D., Munn, A., Meikle, W., Eds.; Royal Zoological Society of New South Wales: Mosman, Australia, 2008; pp. 49–51.

35. Inwood, D.; Catanchin, H.; Coulson, G. Roo town slow down: A community-based kangaroo management plan for Anglesea, Victoria. In *Too Close for Comfort: Contentious Issues in Human-Wildlife Encounters*; Lunney, D., Munn, A., Meikle, W., Eds.; Royal Zoological Society of New South Wales: Mosman, Australia, 2008; pp. 1–8.

36. King, W.J.; Wilson, M.E.; Allen, T.; Festa-Bianchet, M.; Coulson, G. A capture technique for free-ranging eastern grey kangaroos (*Macropus giganteus*) habituated to humans. *Aust. Mammal.* **2011**, *33*, 47–51.

37. Clutton-Brock, T.H.; Sheldon, B.C. Individuals and populations: The role of long term, individual-based studies of animals in ecology and evolutionary biology. *Trends Ecol. Evol.* **2010**, *25*, 562–573.

38. Mulder, R.A.; Guay, J.-P.; Wilson, M.; Coulson, G. Citizen science: Recruiting residents for studies of tagged urban wildlife. *Wildl. Res.* **2010**, *37*, 440–446.

39. Cripps, J.; Beveridge, I.; Coulson, G. The efficacy of anthelmintic drugs against nematodes infecting free-ranging eastern grey kangaroos, *Macropus giganteus*. *J. Wildl. Dis.* **2013**, *49*, 535–544.

40. Wilson, M.E.; Coulson, G.; Shaw, G.; Renfree, M.B. Deslorelin implants in free-ranging female eastern grey kangaroos (*Macropus giganteus*): Mechanism of action and contraceptive efficacy. *Wildl. Res.* **2013**, *40*, 403–412.

41. Gélin, U.; Wilson, M.E.; Coulson, G.M.; Festa-Bianchet, M. Offspring sex, current and previous reproduction affect feeding behavior in wild eastern grey kangaroos. *Anim. Behav.* **2013**, *86*, 885–891.

42. *Census of Population and Housing. Economic Development, City of Greater Geelong*; Australian Bureau of Statistics: Belconnen, Australia, 2001.

43. Holdgate, G.R.; Smith, T.A.G.; Gallagher, S.J.; Wallace, M.W. Geology of coal-bearing Palaeogene sediments, onshore Torquay Basin, Victoria. *Aust. J. Earth Sci.* **2001**, *48*, 657–679.

44. Kirkpatrick, T.H. Studies of the Macropodidae in Queensland. 2. Age estimation in the grey kangaroo, the red kangaroo, the eastern wallaroo and the red-necked wallaby, with notes on dental abnormalities. *Qld. J. Agric. Anim. Sci.* **1965**, *22*, 301–317.

45. Ditchkoff, S.S.; Saalfeld, S.T.; Gibson, C.J. Animal behavior in urban ecosystems: Modifications due to human-induced stress. *Urban. Ecosyst.* **2006**, *9*, 5–12.

46. Adderton Herbert, C. Long-acting contraceptives: A new tool to manage overabundant kangaroo populations in nature reserves and urban areas. *Aust. Mammal.* **2004**, *26*, 67–74.

47. Wilson, M.E.; Coulson, G. Unpublished data, 2014.

48. Porter, W.F.; Underwood, H.B. *Contraception & Deer: The Irondequoit Report*; Roosevelt Wild Life Station: Syracuse, NY, USA, 2001.

49. van Dijk, A.I. J.M.; Beck, H.E.; Crosbie, R.S.; de Jeu, R.A. M.; Liu, Y.Y.; Podger, G.M.; Timbal, B.; Viney, N.R. The Millennium Drought in southeast Australia (2001–2009): Natural and human causes and implications for water resources, ecosystems, economy, and society. *Water Resour. Res.* **2013**, *49*, 1040–1057.

50. Kirkpatrick, T.H.; McEvoy, J.S. Studies of Macropodidae in Queensland. 5. Effects of drought on reproduction in the grey kangaroo (*Macropus giganteus*). *Qld. J. Agric. Anim. Sci.* **1966**, *23*, 339–442.

51. Banks, P.B.; Newsome, A.E.; Dickman, C.R. Predation by red foxes limits recruitment in populations of eastern grey kangaroos. *Aust. Ecol.* **2000**, *25*, 283–291.

52. Jarman, P.J; Taylor, R.J. Ranging of eastern grey kangaroos and wallaroos on a New England pastoral property. *Aust. Wildl. Res.* **1983**, *10*, 33–38.

53. Jaremovic, R.V.; Croft, D.B. Comparison of techniques to determine eastern grey kangaroo home range. *J. Wildl. Manage.* **1987**, *51*, 921–930.

54. Moore, B.D.; Coulson, G.; Way, S. Habitat selection by adult female eastern grey kangaroos. *Wildl. Res.* **2002**, *29*, 439–445.

55. Viggers, K.L.; Hearn, J.P. The kangaroo conundrum: Home range studies and implications for management. *J. Appl. Ecol.* **2005**, *42*, 99–107.

56. Grund, M.D.; McAninch, J.B.; Wiggers, E.B. Seasonal movements and habitat use of female white-tailed deer associated with an urban park. *J. Wildl. Manage.* **2002**, *66*, 123–130.

57. Storm, D.J.; Nielsen, C.K.; Schauber, E.M.; Woolf, A. Space use and survival of white-tailed deer in an exurban landscape. *J. Wildl. Manage.* **2007**, *71*, 1170–1176.

58. MacFarlane, A.M.; Coulson, G. Sexual segregation in Australian marsupials. In *Sexual Segregation in Vertebrates*; Ruckstuhl, K.E., Neuhaus, H., Eds.; Cambridge University Press: Cambridge, UK, 2005; pp. 254–279.

59. ACT Kangaroo Advisory Committee. *Living With Eastern Grey Kangaroos in the ACT—Public Land*; Third Report to the Minister for the Environment, Land And Planning; Publications and Public Communication for Environment ACT: Canberra, Australia, 1997.

60. Coulson, G.M. Road-kills of macropods on a section of highway in central Victoria. *Aust. Wildl. Res.* **1982**, *9*, 21–26.

61. Coulson, G. Male bias in road-kills of macropods. *Wildl. Res.* **1997**, *23*, 21–25.

62. McAlpine, C.A.; Grigg, G.C.; Mott, J.J.; Sharma, P. Influence of landscape structure on kangaroo abundance in a disturbed semi-arid woodland of Queensland. *Rangel. J.* **1999**, *21*, 104–134.

63. Hennessy, C.A.; Dubach, J.; Gehrt, S.D. Long-term pair bonding and genetic evidence for monogamy among urban coyotes (*Canis latrans*). *J. Mammal.* **2012**, *93*, 732–742.

64. Cripps, J.; Beveridge, I.; Ploeg, R.; Coulson, G. Experimental manipulation reveals few subclinical impacts of a parasite community in juvenile kangaroos. *IJP-PAW* **2014**, *3*, 88–94.

65. Morishita, E.; Itao, J.; Sasaki, K.; Higuchi, H. Movements of crows in urban areas, based on PHS tracking. *Global Env. Res.* **2003**, *7*, 181–192.

66. Grinder, M.I.; Krausman, P.R. Home range, habitat use, and nocturnal activity of coyotes in an urban environment. *J. Wildl. Manage.* **2001**, *65*, 887–898.

7

Cows Come Down from the Mountains before the (M_w = 6.1) Earthquake Colfiorito in September 1997; A Single Case Study

Cristiano Fidani [1,2,*], Friedemann Freund [3,4,5] and Rachel Grant [6]

[1] Osservatorio Sismico "Andrea Bina", Borgo XX Giugno 74, 06121 Perugia, Italy

[2] Central Italy Electromagnetic Network (CIEN), Via Fosso del Passo 6, 63847 San Procolo, Fermo, Italy

[3] Ames Research Center, National Aeronautics and Space Administration (NASA), Earth Science Division, Code SGE, Moffett Field, CA 94035, USA; E-Mail: friedemann.t.freund@nasa.gov

[4] Department of Physics, San Jose State University, San Jose, CA 95192, USA

[5] Carl Sagan Center, SETI Institute, 189 Bernardo Ave., Mountain View, CA 94043, USA

[6] Department of Life Sciences, Anglia Ruskin University, East Rd., Cambridge, CB1 1PT, UK; E-Mail: Rachel.grant@anglia.ac.uk

* Author to whom correspondence should be addressed; E-Mail: c.fidani@virgilio.it.

Simple Summary: Recent reports from several countries such as China, Italy and Japan support the existence of strange animal behaviour before strong earthquakes. However, the stimuli to which animals are sensitive preceding seismic activity are still not completely understood. Here we report the case of a herd of cows (reported by an entire village) leaving the hill pasture and descending near to the village streets two days before a strong earthquake.

Abstract: The September–October 1997 seismic sequence in the Umbria–Marche regions of Central Italy has been one of the stronger seismic events to occur in Italy over the last thirty years, with a maximum magnitude of M_w = 6.1. Over the last three years, a collection of evidence was carried out regarding non-seismic phenomena, by interviewing local residents using a questionnaire. One particular observation of anomalous animal behaviour, confirmed by many witnesses, concerned a herd of cows, which descended from a mountain close to the streets of a village near the epicentre, a few days before the main shock. Testimonies were collected using a specific questionnaire including data on earthquake lights, spring variations, human diseases, and irregular animal behaviour. The questionnaire was compiled after the L'Aquila earthquake in 2009, and was based upon past historical earthquake observations. A possible explanation for the cows' behavior—local air ionization caused by stress-activated positive holes—is discussed.

Keywords: animal behaviour; earthquakes; positive holes; air ionization; cows

---

1. Introduction

Unusual animal behaviour prior to earthquakes has been observed for millennia [1], but until recently, there appeared to be no plausible explanation. Freund [2] presented a unified theory of non-seismic earthquake precursors, proposed on the basis of stress-activated positive hole charge carriers. It is likely that at least some of the observations of unusual pre-earthquake animal behaviour can be traced back to this underlying geophysical process. Other possible causes are the release of gases, such as CO, from the future epicentre [3], charged aerosol production [4], sound and vibrations [5], electric [6] and magnetic [7] field influences, ultra-low and extra-low-frequency electromagnetic effects [8,9]. It should be remembered that species-typical behaviours can be triggered by a variety of stimuli not necessarily related to earthquakes [10] and that sometimes animal behaviour anomalies reported by the public may actually not be abnormal behaviour [11]. Often much of the behaviour resembles that reported before other geophysical events, such as thunderstorms [12], or volcanic eruptions [13]. Animal behavior is very variable, even within the same species [14]. Finally, as there are geophysical differences between earthquakes [15], unusual animal behaviour is observed before some earthquakes but not others.

With this in mind, in this communication we present several incidences of unusual behaviour of cattle and also describe a previously unpublished observation of unusual cow behaviour prior to the Umbria-Marche earthquake ($M_w = 6.1$) of September 26, 1997. An evaluation in terms of the theory of positive holes leading to air ionization as proposed by Freund et al. [16] was applied to the Colfiorito tectonic structure in Central Italy, where the strong earthquake struck.

The Colfiorito area is a closed extensional basin system located on the Apennines watershed and surrounded by valleys that are deeply incised into the Mesozoic–Cenozoic bedrock (Figure 1). The basin floor is at an elevation of 800 m whereas the level of river incision in nearby valleys rapidly decreases to 400 m within a few kilometres of the basin. Lacustrine and alluvial deposits containing remains of Lower Pleistocene mammal fauna [17] are exposed for 100 m in thickness in the central and southern parts of the basin. Surface geological data and seismic reflection profiles have clearly pointed out that the area of Colfiorito is structurally dominated by N–S and NNW–SSE trending macro-anticlines. Colfiorito plain is bounded to the NE by an active normal fault system [18] that ruptured during the 1997 Umbria-Marche earthquake sequence [19]. Despite the different interpretations given to the surface ruptures observed after the main shocks, the fault geometry revealed by seismological, geodetic, and field data [20,21] is consistent with the longer-term Quaternary evolution of the area. In particular, radar interferometry and GPS data showed several tens of centimetres of seismic subsidence in the hangingwall of the fault system bounding the basin [22], and surface ruptures of a few cm in amplitude were found after the earthquake along previously-mapped fault scarps at the foot of mountain fronts bounding the Quaternary basin [23].

The seismic sequence that affected the Umbria–Marche region (Central Italy) in the period September 1997–April 1998 caused the loss of 12 lives and severe damage to ca. 300 localities. Three main events took place at less than 10 km depth: two on September 26, 1997, (1) M_w = 5.8 and (2) M_w = 6.1, and one on October 14, 2007, (3) M_w = 5.6; indicated by red circles in Figure 1.

Figure 1. Colfiorito Basin. The red arrows in the left-hand box indicate cow movements, while red circles indicate the stronger shocks and blue circles indicate meteorological stations at Serravalle (1), Gelagna Alta (2), Pié del Sasso (3) and Bagnara (4) (the Nocera Umbra station is outside of the map to the west near Bagnara). A section of the Basin in the left-hand box is shown in red, it is represented in the right-hand box with the positions of the main shock and aftershocks along the normal fault plane in red; Mount Maggio is behind Mount Prefoglio, after Barchi [24].

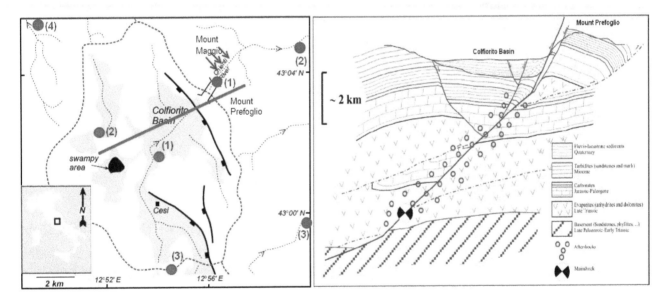

2. Methods

The L'Aquila earthquake has shown that the public is able to observe a large number of phenomena for which there were no available instruments at the time of the quake, including unusual animal behaviour [25]. The people of L'Aquila clearly remembered their observations for many months and in many cases they remembered observations from previous earthquakes. Hence, a collection of data was carried out relative to a strong earthquake which occurred some time before L'Aquila, that of Colfiorito.

Testimonies of unusual behaviour of wild and domestic animals were collected around Colfiorito Plain in connection with the September 1997 earthquake. The observations were collected in the months of September–October 2010, August–September 2011, May-August and October–November 2012, January and April 2013. People reported strange animal behaviour which had occurred in September 1997, *i.e.*, more than 13 years ago. It is possible that people's memories are inaccurate and data may be unreliable after such as long period of time. However, it is also remarkable that so many people independently remembered and commented on the particular observation presented here. A questionnaire was used to obtain information on sightings of earthquake lights, with a small section on animal behaviour anomalies. The questionnaire was initially used to collect information relative to the L'Aquila earthquake in 2009 [26] (the full text can be downloaded from supplementary material [26]). Here, the section concerning animals is shown:

Did you observe strange behaviour on the part of animals?

If yes, please describe the places, times and conditions:

    55) Sudden death of domestic or stray animals?

    56) Yelping of dogs?

    57) Neighing of horses?

    58) Unexplainable appearance of ants?

    59) Abundant appearance of worms?

    60) Unexplainable appearance of snakes or frogs?

    61) Unexplainable appearance of mice?

    62) Unexplainable behaviour of chickens?

    63) Unexplainable behaviour of fish?

    64) Nervous behaviour of farming livestock?

    65) Sighting of rare animals?

    66) Disappearance of birds?

    67) Other strange animal behaviour? Please describe:

    Other, please describe:

This same questionnaire was used with the population of the regions of Umbria and Marche, affected by the strong earthquake of Colfiorito in September 1997. Questionnaires were not distributed on paper to the population but carried out by face to-face interviews, allowing as much information as possible to be collected [27]. A total of 94 people were interviewed in the Umbria-Marche region.

3. Observations and Results

3.1. Cows

The observation on which we report here, was made in Serravalle del Chienti, a village located a few kilometers north-east of the earthquake epicentre of September 26, 1997, $M_w = 6.1$. Nineteen out of 94 people were interviewed in Serravalle, and of these, 17 reported behaviour which they considered anomalous, *i.e.*, cows descending to near the village before the earthquake. The cows were grazing on the top of Monte Maggio, located north of Serravalle, which is the village in a valley that separates it from Mount Prefoglio, see Figure 2. The cows are always let loose on the pastures (at Monte Maggio 1236 m) every summer. They return to their barn when the snow comes, usually at the end of November or beginning of December. The villagers know that the cows normally stay in the pasture area and do not leave it all summer. Two days before the main shock, however, the herd of cows was sighted near to the village of Serravalle del Chienti in the clearings above the highway 77 at

700 m. About 60 cows, the entire herd, had descended from the mountain (Figure 2) and into the town itself, which is a highly unusual behaviour, although all cows seemed to be in good health. The cows were seen by all the inhabitants of the village a few days before the earthquake. The reports confirmed that cattle descended from the mountain and stood in the area above the highway 77 for 4–5 days, after which time, the cattle went back up the mountain. The interviewees who observed the cows were asked if this has ever occurred again since the earthquake. Some people reported seeing the cows descending from the mountain at other times, such as when there was a sudden change in the weather, in particular the arrival of very bad weather or heavy snow. For this reason weather data were analyzed to rule out unusual weather as a cause of the cow movements.

Figure 2. A Google Earth map of the Colfiorito Basin, red arrow indicates cow movements.

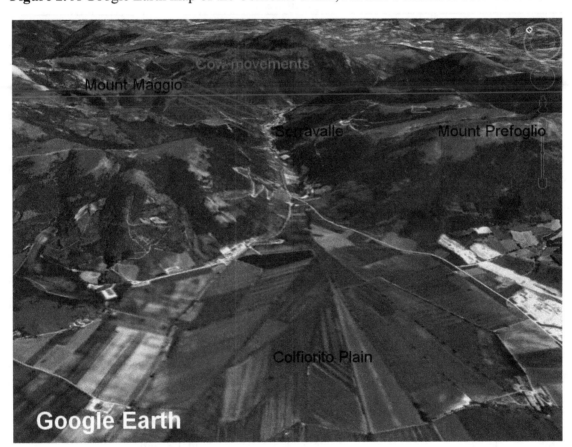

3.2. Other Macroscopic Anomalies

A systematic literature search was carried out using scientific databases (ISI Web of Knowledge and Google Scholar), to find unusual behaviour of free ranging cattle. The search terms used were "cow" OR "cattle" AND "unusual behaviour/behaviour" which brought up more than 1000 documents, most of which were not relevant. Many of the observations of unusual behaviour of cattle prior to earthquakes related to restrained animals in domestic situations, and the general reaction was panic and attempts to escape. These were not included. Eight observations were found which are summarised in Table 1. We have also included in this table the 26 September 1997 Colfiorito earthquake of $M_w = 6.1$, which was preceded by a strong foreshock of $M_w = 5.8$.

Table 1. A summary of reports of unusual behaviour in free ranging cattle.

Behaviour	When behaviour occurred	Earthquake or possible explanation	Source
Cattle move to higher ground			
Cattle move to higher pastures	Few hours before earthquake and tsunami	27 March 1964, M = 8.7 Prince William Sound, Alaska. Offshore earthquake leading to tsunami flooding low lying meadows.	Engle, 1965 [28]
Cattle move to high ground	Before tsunami	26 December 2004. M = 9.1 Off shore earthquake off the coast of Aceh, Indonesia leading to flooding of low lying areas	Kelman et al. 2004 [29]
Cattle come down from hills			
Cattle come down from the hills	"shortly" before earthquake	18 April 1903. M = 8.3 San Fransisco, USA,	Lawson, 1908 [30]
Cattle come down from the hills	2 days prior to earthquake	26 September 1997. Colfiorito Earthquake of M = 5.8 (00:33 GMT) and M = 6.1 (09:40 GMT)	Fidani, 2013 [31]
Cattle leave high pastures on volcano	Just before volcano erupted	29 July 1968. Arenal Volcano erupted, Costa Rica	Anderson, 1973 [32]
Other unusual behaviour observed			
Cows enter suburb of major city	2 days prior to earthquake. Bukit Jalil, KL, Malaysia. April 9, 2012	11 April 2012. M = 8.6 Of the coast of Sumatra	Word Press, 2012 [33]
Hundreds of cows suddenly sit down in unison	Minutes before earthquake	22 February 2011. M = 6.3 Christchurch, New Zealand.	Whitehead and Ulusoy, 2013 [34]
28 cows die after falling over cliff	Lauterbrunnen, Switzerland	August 2009. No earthquake, thought to be related to violent thunderstorms	MailOnline, 2009 [35]
Cows exhibit no unusual behaviour			
Cows exhibit no unusual behaviour		16 December 2008. M = 4.7 Skåne, Sweden. Small earthquake, with different process to those expected to produce large scale ionisation	Haines, 2009 [36]

Meteorological data were retrieved from the Hydrogeological Annals of the Marche Region [37] and Umbria Region [38], from five stations around Colfiorito, (blue circles in Figure 1), and data were recorded with daily samples, (Figure 3a). Temperatures were reported in Figure 3b from the two stations closest to the epicentre. Gas emission data were retrieved from publications [39–42] and were also reported by the people filling in the questionnaires [31].

Figure 3. Rain data from the five meteorological stations. (**a**) rain data after September 22 were lost from Serravalle as it was strongly damaged by the quake; minimum and maximum daily temperatures recorded at Nocera Umbra, in red, and at Foligno, in blue, meteorological stations (**b**) temperature data after September 24 were lost from Nocera Umbra as it was strongly damaged by the quake; the main shock time is indicated by a black vertical line.

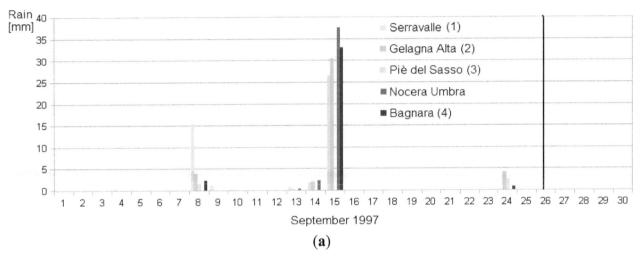

(a)

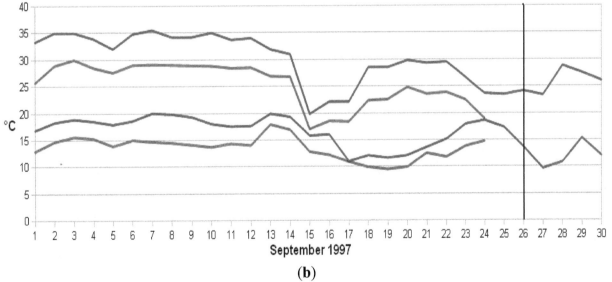

(b)

Earthquake lights (EQL) were also recorded in the vicinity. For example [31], light flashes were observed from Annifo above this village, few kilometers west of Monte Maggio, about two days before the main shock; and red sky was observed during the darkness from the Taverne village in the Colfiorito Plain, a few kilometers south of Monte Maggio, the night of the earthquake after the first shock at 2:33 LT (M_w = 5.8) and several hours before the main shock at 11:42 LT (M_w = 6.1). EQL are common phenomena for moderate earthquakes in Central Italy. The first collection of EQL data reported fire columns and red sky prior to many strong historical earthquakes [43] and contained the first classification based on shapes, colours, and time. Frederic Montandon proposed a revised classification, which reduced Galli's number of EQL types from nine to five [44]. The first EQLs were photographically documented in 1966 along with a report containing numerous testimonials during an earthquake swarm near Matsushiro [45]. A review of observations has highlighted the well-established existence of luminous phenomena plus proposed theories [46]. A recent study on positive charge generation in igneous rocks opened the way to explaining luminous and other phenomena in a single coherent physical model [47]. Charge accumulations at asperities in the crust can produce corona discharges accompanied by the emission of light [48].

4. Theoretical Background

Rocks are generally good insulators. However, all rocks in the Earth's deeper crust contain minerals, with point defects that had not been previously recognized. These defects are peroxy links such as $O_3Si/^{OO}\backslash SiO_3$ replacing the usual $O_3Si/^{O}\backslash SiO_3$ bonds. They are unusual because, in their normal state, they are dormant and electrically inactive. However, when rocks are stressed, peroxy links break and release mobile, positive electronic charge carriers. These are defect electrons in the O^{2-} sub-lattice, chemically equivalent to O^- in a matrix of O^{2-}, known as positive holes and symbolized by $h^{\bullet}$ [49]. Positive holes are highly mobile. They are capable of flowing out of the stressed rock volume in which they were activated, spreading into the surrounding less stressed or unstressed rocks. They travel fast and far, tens of kilometers through the Earth's crust, prior to large earthquakes maybe as much as hundreds of kilometers. As the $h^{\bullet}$ flow, they form electric currents in the Earth's crust, often transient current pulses, but less frequently persistent fluctuation trains lasting hours or longer and tens to hundreds of thousands amperes strong [50]. When these $h^{\bullet}$ currents fluctuate, they emit electromagnetic (EM) radiation, of which the ultra low frequencies (ULF) and extremely low frequencies (ELF) can be transmitted through tens of kilometers of rocks and detected at the Earth's surface. When the $h^{\bullet}$ arrive at the Earth's surface, situations arise, which may be very relevant to the response of animals.

As their name suggests, positive holes are positive charges. Inside the Earth they repel each other electrostatically and "try" to get away from each other as far as they can. The Earth's surface is as far as they can go, but even at the Earth's surface the $h^{\bullet}$ will seek out topographic high points. They accumulate just below the surface, forming a positive charge layer with thickness d, generally some tens of nanometers. This subsurface charge layer is associated with a surface potential, V, typically on the order of 2–3 V.

As the rocks deep below around the hypocenter of the future earthquake, experience increasing levels of stress, ever more $h^{\bullet}$ charge carriers are activated. They will find their way to the surface and contribute to the build-up of the subsurface charge layer. The more $h^{\bullet}$ arrive, the more they compress the subsurface charge layer. Of special interest is the electric field E associated with such surface charge layers.

The electric field E is defined as potential V divided by the thickness d, E = V/d. If V reaches, say, 2 V and the thickness d of the $h^{\bullet}$ subsurface charge layer is, say, 100 nm (1×10^{-6} cm), the E field at the surface will be on the order of 2,000,000 V/cm. As the thickness d of the subsurface charge layer shrinks with the arrival of more $h^{\bullet}$, the E field grows. For instance, if V becomes 3 V and d shrinks to 30 nm (3×10^{-7} cm), the E field will be on the order of 10,000,000 V/cm. Under the effect of such steep E fields, even when they are microscopic and only act at very short range, air molecules become polarized in contact with the surface—so much so that they can lose an electron to the surface and become ionized. During this process, known as field-ionization, the air molecules, most likely O_2, transfer an electron to an $h^\bullet$ in the surface, *i.e.*, to an O^-, converting it to O^{2-}:

$$O^-|_{surface} + O_2|_{air} => O^{2-}|_{surface} + O_2^+|_{air} \qquad (1)$$

Equation (1) describes a process that causes the near-surface air to become laden with positive airborne ions such as O_2^+. All it takes is a sufficiently large number of $h^\bullet$ charge carriers, stress-activated deep below, coming to the Earth's surface above the future earthquake hypocenter and form subsurface charge layers that generate the steepest E fields. Since the $h^\bullet$ repel each other electrostatically, they will seek out the higher elevations. Hence, if an earthquake is preparing to strike in a mountainous area, the reaction described by Equation (1) is most likely to start in the hills.

Figure 4. Laboratory set-up to measure surface potential (**a**) and air ionization (**b**) during stressing a block of rock [16].

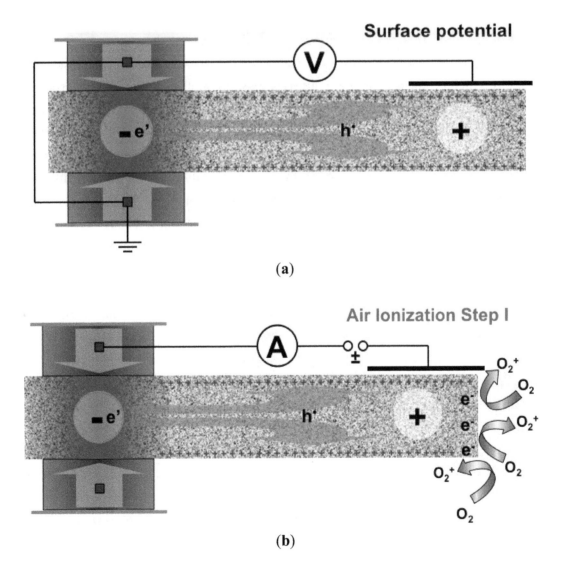

(a)

(b)

Using an experimental set-up as depicted in Figure 4a it has been shown that, when a block of rock is mechanically stressed at one end, a positive surface potential develops at the other end that can be recorded by a voltmeter attached to a metal plate held 2 mm above the rock surface. Upon stressing the rock the surface potential rapidly increases to values around 2–3 V. Upon further loading of the end of the rock, the air in contact with the rock surface at the far end becomes positively ionized as indicated in Figure 4b [16]. This can be recorded by replacing the voltmeter in Figure 4a with an ammeter and insert a battery into the circuit so that the metal plate, held 2 mm above the rock surface, now acts as an ion collector. The number of positive airborne ions generated on the surface of a chunk of bare rock at moderate loads, typically less than 50% of the fracture strength, can reach values on the order of 10^6–10^7 cm^{-2}·sec^{-1}. Though we don't know yet how these laboratory ionization production rates (in number of ions produced per unit surface) translate into actual air ion concentrations (number of ions per unit volume) in the field, data from Japan [51] indicate that positive air ion concentrations at ground level can be 2–3 orders of magnitude higher than the "fair weather" ion content, typically 200 cm^{-3}, which is primarily due to cosmic rays and radon decay products [52]. Field data recorded by air ionization sensors collocated with the ULF search coil magnetometers of the QuakeFinder stations along the San Andreas Fault system in California and along the subduction zone in southern Peru have recorded massive pre-earthquake air ionization, often lasting for hours, producing predominantly or exclusively positive air ions [53,54].

It should also be noted that the generation of positive airborne ions is only Step I of the air ionization. When more h˙ arrive due to the continuing build-up of tectonic stresses deep below, Stage II can set in which produces even more air ions, but now both positive and negative. The reason is that, with further increase in the number of h˙ in the subsurface charge layer, the surface potential increases and the thickness of the surface/subsurface charge layer decreases. If the potential V reaches, say, 3 V, and the thickness d is reduced to, say, 6 nm, the E field would reach values on the order of 50,000,000 V/cm. Such high fields, even though they may act only over micrometer distances or less, can accelerate free electrons, which are always present in the ambient air due to ionization by cosmic rays and radon, to such high velocities that they begin to impact-ionize air molecules in their path. Such impact ionization events, which are likely to take place above sharp points, edges and corners, produce avalanches of electrons and positive ions, albeit in tiny air volumes, which trigger corona discharges.

Indeed, tiny, rapid-fire 1.5 millisecond light flashes originating at the edges and corners of blocks of rock have been recorded in laboratory experiments as schematically shown in Figure 5 [16], generating bursts of free electrons and positive ions in roughly equal numbers. There seems to be no study cited in the literature that looked at the response to animals to an increase in the total air ion content, both positive and negative in equal proportion, compared to selectively positive air ionization. Animals might be sensitive to an overall increase in air ion concentrations but probably less so than to increases in selective positive air ionization. Furthermore, reaching the surface the charge cloud causes dielectric breakdown at the air-rock interface, i.e., corona discharges, accompanied by the emission of light and high frequency electromagnetic radiation [16]. The light emissions observed at Colfiorito could have originated for the same physical process. Therefore this paper provides a small piece of evidence for Freund's [55] unified theory of earthquake precursors.

Figure 5. Schematic representation of the 2-step air ionization that has been demonstrated in laboratory experiments during stressing of rocks [16].

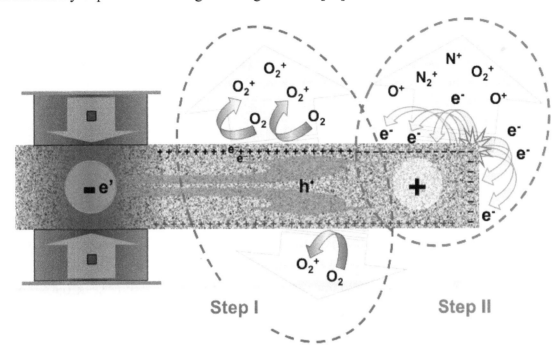

A parallel effect might have to be considered. As with any corona discharge in air, the flashes do emit light, which spans a broad spectrum over the VIS and UV regions, including "hard" UV. The hard UV portion will produce ozone, O_3, and other reactive gases such as nitrous oxides, to which animals might also respond [56].

5. Discussion

It has been speculated that unusual animal movements could be caused by sound and ultrasound, such as before the Sumatra 2004 tsunami [57]. Sounds and explosions were also heard by the Colfiorito population, but these occurred months before the main shock [31] and no cow movements were observed at that time. The arrival of P waves could provide a possible causal link to many forms of unusual animal behaviour [58]. However P waves arrive only a few seconds before S waves, while the cows migrated down from the mountain two days before the quake, on September 24, 1997. The possibility of a P wave effect from a strong foreshock can also be ruled out, as the only foreshock (of magnitude 4) struck September 4, 1997, with no unusual cow movements in evidence. It is also highly unlikely that cows in Western Europe would move to avoid a predator. Cows are large animals and of course do have predators, but these are mainly large carnivores such as lions, panthers *etc.* that are not found in Central Italy. There are wolves and bears in some national parks of central Italy but they are few in number (having been reintroduced as a conservation effort) and they would not target a whole herd of adult cows.

Meteorological data indicate that the cattle movements were not caused by unusual weather. Figure 3a shows that abundant rainfall occurred on September 15 and slight rainfall on September 24. Temperatures reported in Figure 3b were within the norms of the season, which was verified by calculating weekly averages at the Foligno station where data had been available for 20 years.

Maximum daily temperatures did not exceed two standard deviations, whereas minimum daily temperatures did not drop below two standard deviations. Both meteorological stations were not on the Colfiorito Plain, but in Nocera Umbra and Foligno at distances of 10 km and 20 km from the epicenter respectively. An intense and concentrated episode of evaporation reported on some occasions [1] and demonstrated in certain conditions [59], cannot be excluded. If, however, evaporation occurred it would not have been due to weather conditions, which usually affect regions much greater that the thermometric station distances from the epicentre considered here.

Positive airborne ions have long been known to have a strong physiological effect on animals and humans [60,61]. Therefore, it should not come as a surprise that animals on the ground and in the air, when exposed to high levels of positive airborne ions, would respond in ways which would minimize their exposure. In the case of the cows that left their pasture on top of Monte Maggio prior to the September 26 earthquake to seek refuge in Serravalle del Chienti, the unusual interruption of their summer grazing routine appears to be consistent with the known physics that controls the flow of stress-activated h⋅ charge carriers in an area of impending earthquake activity. Since the h⋅ charge carriers repel each other in the rocks as they spread toward the surface and "seek out" topographic heights, the air ionization process will begin with positive airborne ions generated massively on hilltops and other high elevation points.

The fact that the herd of cows left its high-lying summer grazing grounds to seek refuge in the valley is consistent with the expected elevation-dependent concentration gradient of positive airborne ions. As more and more stress-activated h⋅ charges arrive from below, the positive air ionization will probably spread to lower elevations, including the valleys. There is little recent research on the effects of positive ions on biological systems, however, research conducted in the 1960s and 1970s showed that positive air ions cause irritability and impaired motor abilities probably due to the fact that positive ions increase serotonin levels [61,62]. High levels of serotonin can also be caused by some antidepressant medication, so there has been much recent research on the dangers of high serotonin which can lead to serotonin syndrome, a potentially fatal condition. Symptoms of serotonin syndrome in humans include confusion, agitation, tremors or involuntary movements, akathisia (moderate to severe restlessness), hyperactivity, anxiety, and physiological symptoms such as hypertension and diarrhea, hypothermia [63–65].

Other pre-earthquake non-seismic phenomena may potentially have a noticeable effect on biological systems. In addition to the release of massive amounts of air ions, other gases have been reported to be released pre-seismically. One of the most toxic gases most likely to affect organisms is carbon monoxide [66]. Preseismic and coseismic geochemical variations were detected in some gas vents and natural springs during the 1997 seismic crisis in central Italy, interpreted as rate variations possibly due to crustal permeability changes [39]. Dissolved gases at nearby springs exhibited a slight enrichment of dissolved CO_2 and CH_4 after the main shock [40]. It has been suggested that increased CO_2 pressure triggered aftershock activity by significantly reducing the effective normal stress [41].

CO data were collected only after September 1997 in Central Italy [42] and there are no data relative to the period of August–September 1997.

Carbon monoxide is highly toxic because it deprives the body of vital oxygen. Carbon monoxide binds preferentially with haemoglobin (the substance which transports oxygen in the blood stream) and prevents the O_2 being carried to the tissues. Carbon monoxide's affinity for haemoglobin is 200 times that of oxygen, meaning that it will bind preferentially even at relatively low concentrations, leading to the formation of carboxyhaemoglobin and shifting the oxyhaemoglobin dissociation curve leftwards. As a result of follow-on reactions in the organism the result is hypoxia which can lead to death of the organism [67,68]. Symptoms of CO poisoning in humans include headache, nausea, and dizziness, confusion, weakness, and in more severe cases, respiratory and cardiac failure and eventually, coma [69].

According to the questionnaire, sulfurous gas emissions in the Colfiorito area seem to have been concentrated in the valley floor, thus they are unlikely to have been the cause of the unusual cow movements down the mountain.

Although avoidance tests have not yet been specifically carried out with positive air ions, carbon monoxide and sulfurous gases, animals will generally seek to avoid and move away from harmful and toxic substances in their environment. For example, animals will generally show avoidance responses to pollutants in their environments [70], so much so that many organisms' avoidance responses are used as bioassays for the presence of pollutants [71–73].

5.1. Behaviour of Domestic Cows and other Animals before Earthquakes

The cow (*Bos primigenius*) *is* a domesticated species of ungulate with a long association with humans for the purpose of providing meat and milk [74]. Cows are a species of animal that tends to follow a predictable routine, not generally deviating from it [74]. Cows have been reported for centuries to exhibit strange behaviour prior to earthquakes [1]. Twenty to thirty hours before the Lisbon earthquake, November 1, 1755, cattle became very excited. Excessive excitement, panic or vocalization of cattle has been observed before many other earthquakes as well including that in Naples, Italy in 1805; Fruili, Italy on May 6, 1976 and the 1907 Karatagh earthquake in the border area between Uzbekistan and Tajikistan. Cattle have been reported to refuse to enter their stalls (Tangshan earthquake of May 25, 1970), to behave aggressively and to attack each other (Haicheng earthquake of February 4, 1975) [1].

Of interest are the two different types of behaviour exhibited by cows (aggressive or excited, as opposed to simply moving between high and low areas). Domestic animals are often reported to panic and break free of tethers, or to become aggressive, agitated or restless, whereas wild animals are usually reported to leave an area and move somewhere else. In the book on animal behaviour and earthquakes by Tributsch [1], wild animals are reported to show unusual movements, whereas domestic animals mainly show restlessness, aggression and attempts to escape (summarised in Table 2). This could be interpreted as animals moving away from aversive stimuli to other areas, and those prevented from doing so start to panic or attempt to escape. This observation, along with others of cow movements prior to natural disasters, supports the hypothesis [75] that unusual behaviour prior to earthquake is primarily a movement away from toxic or aversive stimuli. As discussed, in terrestrial animals, these are likely to be gasses such as CO released from the fault [3] or high concentrations of positive air ions [16].

Table 2. Summary of Reponses of wild *vs.* domestic/captive animals prior to earthquakes (adapted from Tributsch [1]).

Wild or Unrestrained Animals	Domestic or Captive animals
Birds • behave fearfully or agitated • take to the air en masse • leave the trees, nests or dovecote • vocalising excessively • leave usual habitat • giant flocks seen	**Dogs** • barking, whining or howling excessively • fearfully, agitated or restless • escaped/lost
Rats and/or weasels • fleeing the town or city • appear in packs • leave houses and granaries or other buildings • run around town	**Horses** • behaving fearfully, agitated or restless • stamping, kicking or rolling on the ground. • impossible to ride or refusing to walk • breaking out of halter or tether • vocalising excessively • escaped/lost
Reptiles and amphibians • Snakes leave their burrows in winter/crawl on snowy ground • Snakes seen in large numbers • Turtles jump out of water • Lizards come out of their burrows • Amphibians leave their breeding site	**Domestic birds (Hens/Chickens/Geese)** • refuse to enter coops • behave fearfully or agitated • excessively noisy • Cockerels crow all night long • break out of enclosure or try to escape • escape/lost
Invertebrates • Swarm of bees leave the area • Ants leave holes • Sea cucumbers disappear • Large numbers of earthworms leave the soil • Large numbers of sea urchins appear • Large crab migrations/crabs crawl to shore • Plankton comes to the surface • Large number of flying ants seen • Swarms of millipedes are seen • Sea snakes swim upriver • Lobster and squid caught at surface • Many octopuses in shallow water or acting strangely	**Cattle/pigs/sheep** • behave fearfully or agitated, restless • refuse to enter stalls • vocalising excessively • become aggressive, bite each other • try to break out of enclosures • escape from enclosures/lost **Zoo animals** • behave fearfully, excited or restless • refuse to enter pens or enclosures • try to breakout of enclosures • escape/lost

The literature search and the observation at Colfiorito show that the behaviour of free ranging cows before natural disasters is highly context specific. Cows have been shown to adjust their movements before earthquakes, tsunamis, volcanoes and other natural disasters. Kirschvink [58] discusses the possibility of animals having an evolved seismic escape response. This is plausible if movement to higher or lower ground before natural disasters increased survival chances, leading to a genetic predisposition to avoid stimuli which are reliably linked to future natural hazards. By way of a

Monte-Carlo simulation, Kirschvink [58] shows that rare events such as earthquakes can drive evolutionary change if the consequences are severe enough. However, it is more likely that the more parsimonious explanation is true; animals which behave unusually or adjust their positions before earthquakes are simply moving away from aversive stimuli in their environment. Cows responding to volcanic eruptions and tsunamis may be responding to infrasound, although no evidence exists at present for the stimuli that animals may respond to prior to these particular hazards.

The cause of the stimuli that the animals are avoiding may be different for different earthquakes. For example, Whitehead and Ulusoy [34] suggest that the cows, which changed their body position prior to the Christchurch earthquake, were acting to ease discomfort brought on by exposure to ULF radiation. Ikeya 2004 [76] reports similar behaviour prior to the Gujarat Earthquake in elephants in the nearby Ahmedabad Zoo. Pre-seismic ULF emissions and their likely effects on biological systems provide an additional possible mechanism for the unusual cow movements [9]. Cows are known to align their bodies along the N-S geomagnetic axis. This effect can be disrupted by overhead power lines and their associated magnetic fields [77]. Hence, a possible explanation for unusual cow movements at Colfiorito could be due to ULF magnetic field anomalies, which have been reported to occur before large earthquakes [58]. However, for the Colfiorito earthquake, no convincing evidence for ULF magnetic anomalies in the range of 4–100 mHz was recorded by the geomagnetic station at L'Aquila [78], which is about 80 km from the epicentre of the main shock, making the positive holes hypothesis much more plausible for this particular earthquake.

There is a report of cattle showing no recognizable unusual behaviour before a small earthquake in Sweden on December 16, 2008 [79]. However, this event occurred at 20 km depth and had a magnitude of only M = 4.7, confirming that unusual animal behavior is generally not observed prior to smaller earthquakes M < 5. Furthermore, not every earthquake causes unusual animal behaviour [80], which may be due to differences in geology, focal mechanisms and the specific behaviour of individual animals.

5.2. Possible Cause of Cows Leaving Their Pastures Prior the Colfiorito Earthquake

We have shown that unusual movements of free ranging cattle are not uncommon before earthquakes and other natural hazards (Table 1). The particular case of the Umbria-Marche earthquake, where the tectonic structure of Colfiorito area is well known, suggests the importance of the relative position of Monte Maggio to the fault geometry and position (Figure 6). Even leaving aside the water-saturated sediments in the valleys and the Colfiorito basin, which may inhibit transmission of the electronic charge carriers by ionizing water molecules at the water-rock interface, the density of airborne positive ions will increases on mountain tops. Charge density on the ground is represented by the + symbol density on Figure 6. The earthquake focal mechanism of the Colfiorito fault shows a region of compressive stresses towards Monte Maggio, probably intensifying the flow of charges in that direction. The red lines in Figure 6 represent estimated fair potential lines.

Figure 6. Surface profile extracted from Figure 1b, showing the Colfiorito plain, Monte Prefoglio (and Monte Maggio behind it) relative to the fault geometry which generated the Umbria-Marche earthquake; + symbol represents the charge distribution on the ground surface.

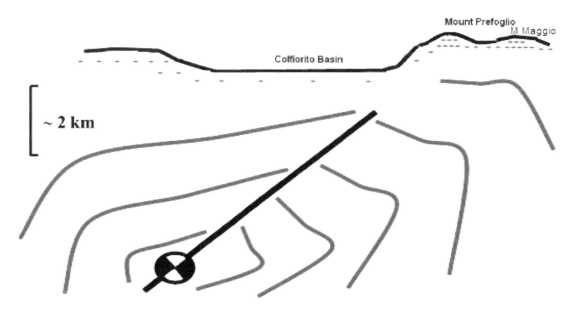

6. Conclusions

Cow movements two days before the Colfiorito, September 26, 1997 Central Italy earthquake, were observed by numerous people in the village of Serravalle del Chienti. As the recorded rainfall and temperature in September 1997 were within seasonal averages, it is unlikely that the cow movements were due to these factors.

The movement of unrestrained animals (such as the cows at Colfiorito) away from their usual habitat which has been observed frequently [1,81] and the excited and agitated way in which they reportedly behave when prevented from leaving an area, may be due to frustration on attempting to escape from the aversive environmental conditions or could be due to the serotonin syndrome. This could be caused by an increase in positive airborne ions due to the arrival, at the ground-to-air interface, of charge carriers, activated deep below the Earth's crust and spread over a wide area surrounding the forthcoming epicentre. The same charge excess could account for luminous effects and earthquake lights, which were also observed in the area.

Acknowledgments

The authors would like to thank the inhabitants of Umbria-Marche for contributing their valuable testimonials. Many thanks also go to Umberto Corridoni, said "Pepper", for his patience and availability to respond to all the questions. The author would also like to thank Maria Teresa Brunetti for her valuable input regarding meteorological observations; Michele Arcaleni and Don Giustino Farnedi for several discussions regarding the manuscript. Finally, thanks go to Antonio Mosciatti for discussing life moments and reporting many observations of children around the Colfiorito earthquake in the book "Mi tremava anche il sogno. L'esperienza del terremoto raccontata dai bambini di Serravalle di Chienti", edited by Ma. Gi., Patti, Messina, December 1997.

Author Contributions

CF collected the testimonials and all data from the Colfiorito area. FF designed the theoretical background. RG carried out the summary of unusual behaviour in free ranging cattle, of domestic/captive response animals prior to earthquakes and discussed the biological part. All authors contributed to the drafting of the overall article.

Conflicts of Interest

The author declares no conflict of interest.

References and Notes

1. Tributsch, H. *When the Snakes Awake: Animals and Earthquake Prediction*; MIT Press: Cambridge, MA, USA, 1984; p. 264.
2. Freund, F.T. Toward a unified solid state theory for pre-earthquake signals. *Acta Geophys.* **2010**, *58*, 719–766.
3. Matteucig, G. *Raccolta di relazioni, comunicazioni ed interventi sul comportamento degli animali in relazione alle variazioni geochimicofisiche ambientali precedenti i sismi*; Assessorato all'Ecologia della Provincia di Napoli: Napoli, Italy, 1985.
4. Tributsch, H. Do aerosol anomalies precede earthquakes? *Nature* **1978**, *276*, 606–608.
5. Gold, T.; Soter, S. Natural explosive noises. *Science* **1979**, *204*, 371–375.
6. Ikeya, M. *Earthquakes and Animals: From Folk Legends to Science;* World Scientific: London, UK, 2004; pp. 90–101.
7. Gawthrop, W.H.; Johnson, R.; Haberman, R.E.; Wyss, M. Preliminary experiments on the behavior of mice before rock failure in the laboratory. In *Abnormal Animal Behavior Prior to Earthquakes, I*; Evernden, J., Ed.; U.S. Geological Survey: Menlo Park, CA, USA, 1976; pp. 205–211.
8. Hayakawa, M. Possible Electromagnetic Effects on Abnormal Animal Behavior before an Earthquake. *Animals* **2013**, *3*, 19–32.
9. Freund, F.; Stolc, V. Nature of Pre-Earthquake Phenomena and their Effects on Living Organisms. *Animals* **2013**, *3*, 513–531.
10. Moore, B.R.; Stuttard, S. Dr. Guthrie and *Felis domesticus* on Tripping over the Cat. *Science* **1979**, *205*, 1031–1033.
11. Grant, R.A.; Conlan, H. Frog Swarms: Earthquake Precursors or False Alarms? *Animals* **2013**, *3*, 962–977.
12. Bufe, C.; Nanewicz, J. Atmospheric electric field observations, animal behaviour and earthquakes. In *Abnormal Animal Behaviour Prior to Earthquakes*; Evernden, J., Eds.; U.S. Geological Survey: Menlo Park, CA, USA, 1976; Volume I.
13. Anderson, C.J. Animals, earthquakes, and eruptions. *Field Mus. Nat. Hist. Bull.* **1973**, *44*, 5–11.
14. Lott, D.F; Hart, B.L.; Verosub, K.L.; Howell, M.W. Is unusual animal behaviour observed before earthquakes? Yes and no. *Geophys. Res. Lett.* **1979**, *6*, 685–687.

15. Lott, D.F.; Hart, B.L.; Howell, M.W. *Animal Behavior and Earthquake Prediction, Final Report*; Contract 91622; U.S. Geological Survey: Reston, VA, USA, 1980.

16. Freund, F.T.; Kulahci, I.; Cyr, G.; Ling, J.; Winnick, M.; Tregloan-Reed, J.; Freund, M.M. Air ionization at rock surface and pre-earthquake signals. *J. Atmos. Sol.-Terr. Phys.* **2009**, *71*, 1824–1834.

17. Coltorti, M.; Albianelli, A.; Bertini, A.; Ficcarelli, G.; Laurenzi, M.A.; Napoleone, G.; Torre, D. The Colle Curti mammal site in the Colfiorito area (Umbria-Marchean Apennine, Italy): Geomorphology, stratigraphy, paleomagnetism and palynology. *Quat. Int.* **1998**, *47–48*, 107–116.

18. Cello, G.; Mazzoli, S.; Tondi, E.; Turco, E. Active tectonics in the central Apennines and possible implications for seismic hazard analysis in peninsular Italy. *Tectonophys.* **1997**, *272*, 43–68.

19. Amato, A.; Azzara, R.; Chiarabba, C.; Cimini, G.B.; Cocco, M.; Di Bona, M.; Margheriti, L. The 1997 Umbria-Marche, Italy, Earthquake Sequence: A first look at the main shocks and aftershocks. *Geophys. Res. Lett.* **1998**, *15*, 2861–2864.

20. Basili, R.; Bosi, V.; Galadini, F.; Galli, P.; Meghraoui, M.; Messina, P.; Moro, M.; Sposato, A. The Colfiorito earthquake sequence of September–October 1997: Surface breaks and seismotectonic implications for the central Apennines (Italy). *J. Earth Eng.* **1998**, *2*, 291–302.

21. Cinti, F.R.; Cucci, L.; Marra, F.; Montone, P. The 1997 Umbria-Marche (Italy) earthquake sequence: Relationship between ground deformation and seismogenic structure. *Geophys. Res. Lett.* **1999**, *26*, 895–898.

22. Stramondo, S. Colfiorito, Italy, earthquakes: Modeled coseismic surface displacements from SAR interferometry and GPS. *Geophys. Res. Lett.* **1999**, *26*, 883–886.

23. D'Agostino, J.A.; Jackson, F.; Dramis, F.; Funiciello, R. Interactions between mantle upwelling, drainage evolution and active normal faulting: An example from the central Apennines (Italy). *Geophys. J. Int.* **2001**, *147*, 475–497.

24. Barchi, M.R. The 1997–98 Umbria-Marche earthquake: "Geological" *vs.* "seismological" faults. Presented at the Workshop of The Colfiorito Earthquake 1997–2007: Ten Years on, Rome, Italy, 8–10 October 2007.

25. Fidani, C. Biological Anomalies around the 2009 L'Aquila Earthquake. *Animals* **2013**, *3*, 693–721.

26. Fidani, C. The earthquake lights (EQL) of the 6 April 2009 Aquila earthquake, in Central Italy. *Nat. Hazards Earth Syst. Sci.* **2010**, *10*, 967–978.

27. Bird, D.K. The use of questionnaires for acquiring information on public perception of natural hazards and risk mitigation—A review of current knowledge and practice. *Nat. Hazards Earth Syst. Sci.* **2009**, *9*, 1307–1325.

28. Engle, E. *Earthquake—The Story of Alaska's Good Friday Disaster*; John Day Company: New York, NY, USA, 1965.

29. Kelman, I.; Spence, R.; Palmer, J.; Petal, M.; Saito, K. Tourists and disasters: Lessons from the 26 December 2004 tsunamis. *J. Coast Conserv.* **2008**, *12*, 105–113.

30. Lawson, A.C. *The California Earthquake of April 18, 1906—Report of the State Earthquake Investigation Commission*; Carnegie Institution of Washington: Washington, DC, USA, 1908; Volume 1, p. 382.

31. Fidani, C. Unpublished data on Colfiorito questionnaire collection, 2013.

32. Anderson, C.J. Animals, Earthquakes and Eruptions. *Bull. Field Mus. Nat. Hist.* **1973**, *44*, 9–11.

33. Strange Animal Behaviour Again: Earthquake In Aceh. *Word Press* 12 April 2012. Available online: https://akupeduliapa.wordpress.com/2012/04/12/strange-animal-behaviour-again-earthquake-in-aceh/ (accessed on 29 May 2014).

34. Whitehead, N.E.; Ulusoy, U.; Asahara, H.; Ikeya, M. Are any public-reported earthquake precursors valid? *Nat. Hazards Earth Syst. Sci.* **2004**, *4*, 463–468.

35. Police baffled as dozens of 'suicidal' cows throw themselves off cliff in the Alps. *Mail Online* 28 August 2009. Available online: http://www.dailymail.co.uk/news/article-1209638/Scientists-baffled-suicidal-cows-throw-cliff-Switzerland.html (accessed on 29 May 2014).

36. Haines, L. Cows can't detect earthquakes: Official Swedish bovine earth-moving experiment ends in disappointment. *The Register - Science* 14 January **2009**. Available online: http://go.theregister.com/tl/1147/-3265/cyber-risk-report-exec-summary.pdf?td=wptl1147tp (accessed on 29 May 2014).

37. Ferretti, M. *Annali Idrologici 1997, Parte Prima*; Centro Funzionale Multirischi per la Meteorologia, L'Idrologia e la Sismologia, Regione Marche, Dipartimento per le Politiche Integrate di Sicurezza e per la Protezione Civile: Ancona, Italy, 2008.

38. Bencivenga, M. *Annali Idrologici 1997, Parte Prima*; Ufficio Idrografico e Mareografico di Roma, Bacini con Foce al Litorale Tirrenico dal Fiora al Lago di Fondi; Istituto Poligrafico dello Stato: Roma, Italy, 2000.

39. Heinicke, J.; Italiano, F.; Lapenna, V.; Martinelli, G.; Nuccio, P.M. Coseimic geochemical variations in some gas emissions of Umbria Region (Central Italy). *Phys. Chem. Earth A* **2000**, *25*, 289–293.

40. Quattrocchi, F.; Pik, R.; Pizzino, L.; Guerra, M.; Scarlato, P.; Angelone, M.; Barbieri, M.; Conti, A.; Marty, B.; Sacchi, E.; Zuppi, G.M.; Lombardi, S. Geochemical changes at the Bagni di Triponzo thermal spring during the Umbria-Marche 1997–1998 seismic sequence. *J. Seismol.* **2000**, *4*, 567–587.

41. Miller, S.A.; Collettini, C.; Chiaraluce, L.; Cocco, M.; Barchi, M.; Kaus, B.J.J. Aftershocks driven by a high-pressure CO_2 source at depth. *Nature* **2004**, *427*, 724–727.

42. Italiano, F.; Martinelli, G.; Bonfanti, P.; Caracausi, A. Long-term (1997–2007) geochemical monitoring of gases from the Umbria-Marche region. *Tectonophysics* **2009**, *476*, 282–296.

43. Galli, I. Raccolta e classificazione di fenomeni luminosi osservati nei terremoti. *Boll. Soc. Sismol. Ital.* **1910**, *XIV*, 221–448 (in Italian).

44. Montandon, F. Lueurs and malaises d'origine seismique. *Geograph. Helvet.* **1948**, *3*, 157–178.

45. Yasui, Y. *A Summary of Studies on Luminous Phenomena Accompanied with Earthquakes*; Dokkyo Medical University: Tokyo, Japan, 1974.

46. Derr, J.S. Earthquake lights: A review of observations and present theories. *Bull. Seism. Soc. Am.* **1973**, *63*, 2177–2187.

47. Freund, F. Charge generation and propagation in rocks. *J. Geodyn.* **2002**, *33*, 545–572.

48. St-Laurent, F.; Derr, J.S.; Freund, F.T. Earthquake lights and the stress-activation of positive hole charge carriers in rocks. *Phys. Chem. Earth* **2006**, *31*, 305–312.

49. Freund, F.T. Pre-Earthquake Signals: Underlying Physical Processes. *J. Asian Earth Sci.* **2011**, *41*, 383–400.

50. Bortnik, J.; Bleier, T.E.; Dunson, C.; Freund, F. Estimating the seismotelluric current required for observable electromagnetic ground signals. *Ann. Geophys.* **2010**, *28*, 1615–1624.

51. Hattori, K.; Wadatsumi, K.; Furuya, R.; Yada, N.; Yamamoto, I.; Ninagawa, K.; Ideta, Y.; Nishihashi, M. Variation of radioactive atmospheric ion concentration associated with large earthquakes. Presented at the American Geophysical Union Fall Meeting, San Francisco, CA, USA, 15–19 December 2008; Abstract S52A-03.

52. Rycroft, M.J.; Harrison, R.G.; Nicoll, K.A.; Mareev, E.A. An Overview of Earth's Global Electric Circuit and Atmospheric Conductivity. *Space Sci. Rev.* **2008**, *137*, 83–105.

53. Bleier, T.; Dunson, C.; Alvarez, C.H.; Freund, F.; Dahlgren, R.P. Correlation of pre-earthquake electromagnetic signals with laboratory and field rock experiments. *Nat. Hazards Earth Syst. Sci.* **2010**, *10*, 1965–1975.

54. Bleier, T.; Dunson, C.; Roth, S.; Heraud, J.A.; Lira, A.; Freund, F.; Dahlgren, R.; Bambery, R.; Bryant, N. Ground-Based and Space-Based Electromagnetic Monitoring for Pre-Earthquake Signals. In *Frontier of Earthquake Prediction Studies*; Hayakawa, M., Ed.; Nihon-Senmontosho-Shuppan Pub. Co.: Tokyo, Japan, 2011.

55. Freund, F. Earthquake Forewarning—A Multidisciplinary Challenge from the Ground up to Space. *Acta Geophys.* **2013**, *61*, 775–807.

56. Ganguly, N.D. Variation in atmospheric ozone concentration following strong earthquakes. *Int. J. Remote Sens.* **2009**, *30*, 349–356.

57. Waltham, T. The Asian Tsunami, 2004. *Mercian Geologist* **2005**, *16*, 99–106.

58. Kirschvink, J.L. Earthquake Prediction by Animals: Evolution and Sensory Perception. *Bull. Seismol. Soc. Am.* **2000**, *90*, 312–323.

59. Pulinets, S. Ionospheric Precursors of Earthquakes; Recent Advances in Theory and Practical Applications. *TAO* **2004**, *15*, 413–435.

60. Krueger, A.P. Are air ions biologically significant? A review of a controversial subject. *Int. J. Biometeorol.* **1972**, *16*, 313–322.

61. Krueger, A.P.; Reed, E.J. Biological impact of small air ions. *Science* **1976**, *193*, 1209–1213.

62. Charry, J.M. Biological effects of air ions: A comprehensive review of laboratory and clinical effects. In *Air Ions: Physical and Biological Aspects*; Charry, J.M., Kavet, R., Eds.; CRC Press: Boca Raton, FL, USA, 1987; pp. 91–150.

63. Bodner, R.A.; Lynch, T.; Lewis, L.; Khan, D. Serotonin syndrome. *Neurology* **1995**, *45*, 219–223.

64. Mason, P.J.; Morris, V.A.; Balcezak, T.J. Serotonin syndrome. Presentation of 2 cases and review of the literature. *Medicine* **2000**, *79*, 201–209.

65. Boyer, E.W.; Shannon, M. The serotonin syndrome. *N. Eng. J. Med.* **2005**, *352*, 1112–1120.

66. Singh, R.P.; Kumar, J.S.; Zlotnicki, J.; Kafatos, M. Satellite detection of carbon monoxide emission prior to the gujarat earthquake of 26 January 2001. *Appl. Geochem.* **2010**, *25*, 585–580.

67. Ernst, A.; Zibrak, J.D. Carbon monoxide poisoning. *N. Eng. J. Med.* **1998**, *339*, 1603–1608.

68. Thom, S.R. Carbon monoxide pathophysiology and treatment. In *Physiology and Medicine of Hyperbaric Oxygen Therapy*; Neuman, T.S., Thom, S.R., Eds.; Saunders Elsevier: Philadelphia, PA, USA, 2008; pp. 321–347.

69. Kao, L.W.; Nañagas, K.A. Carbon monoxide poisoning. *Emerg. Med. Clin. North Am.* **2004**, *22*, 985–1018.

70. Wentsel, R.; McIntosh, A.; McCafferty, W.P.; Atchison, G.; Anderson, V. Avoidance response of midge larvae (*Chironomus tentans*) to sediments containing heavy metals. *Hydrobiologia* **1977**, *55*, 171–175.

71. Black, J.A.; Birge, W.J. *An Avoidance Response Bioassay for Aquatic Pollutants: Completion Report*; University of Kentucky, Water Resources Research Institute: Lexington, KY, USA, 1980.

72. Wiklund, E.A.K.; Börjesson, T.; Wiklund, S.J. Avoidance response of sediment living amphipods to zinc pyrithione as a measure of sediment toxicity. *Mar. Pollut. Bull.* **2006**, *52*, 96–99.

73. Aldaya, M.M.; Lors, C.; Salmon, S.; Ponge, J.F. Avoidance bio-assays may help to test the ecological significance of soil pollution. *Environ. Poll.* **2006**, *140*, 173–180.

74. Albright, J.L.; Arave, C.W. *The Behaviour of Cattle*; CAB Iinternational: Wallingford, UK, 1997.

75. Grant, R.A.; Halliday, T.; Balderer, W.P.; Leuenberger, F.; Newcomer, M.; Cyr, G.; Freund, F.T. Ground water chemistry changes before major earthquakes and possible effects on animals. *Int. J. Env. Res. Pub. Health* **2011**, *8*, 1936–1956.

76. Ikeya, M. *Earthquakes and Animals: From Folk Legends to Science*; World Scientific: London, UK, 2004; p. 295.

77. Burda, H.; Begall, S.; Cervený, J.; Neef, J.; Nemec, P. Extremely low-frequency electromagnetic fields disrupt magnetic alignment of ruminants. *PNAS* **2009**, doi:10.1073/pnas.0811194106.

78. Villante, U.; Vellante, M.; Piancatelli, A. Ultra low frequency geomagnetic field measurements during earthquake activity in Italy (September-October 1997). *Annali di Geofisica* **2001**, *44*, 229–237.

79. Hainer, L. Cows can't detect earthquakes: Official, Swedish bovine earth-moving experiment ends in disappointment. The Register, Posted in Science, 14 January, 2009. Available online: http://www.theregister.co.uk/2009/01/14/cow_earthquake_shocker/ (accessed on 14 May 2014).

80. Buskirk, R.E.; Frohlich, C.L.; Latham, G.V. Unusual animal behavior before earthquakes: A review of possible sensory mechanisms. *Rev. Geophys.* **1981**, *19*, 247–270.

81. Grant, R.A.; Halliday, T. Predicting the unpredictable; evidence of pre-seismic anticipatory behaviour in the common toad. *J. Zool.* **2010**, *281*, 263–271.

Permissions

The contributors of this book come from diverse backgrounds, making this book a truly international effort. This book will bring forth new frontiers with its revolutionizing research information and detailed analysis of the nascent developments around the world.

We would like to thank all the contributing authors for lending their expertise to make the book truly unique. They have played a crucial role in the development of this book. Without their invaluable contributions this book wouldn't have been possible. They have made vital efforts to compile up to date information on the varied aspects of this subject to make this book a valuable addition to the collection of many professionals and students.

This book was conceptualized with the vision of imparting up-to-date information and advanced data in this field. To ensure the same, a matchless editorial board was set up. Every individual on the board went through rigorous rounds of assessment to prove their worth. After which they invested a large part of their time researching and compiling the most relevant data for our readers.

The editorial board has been involved in producing this book since its inception. They have spent rigorous hours researching and exploring the diverse topics which have resulted in the successful publishing of this book. They have passed on their knowledge of decades through this book. To expedite this challenging task, the publisher supported the team at every step. A small team of assistant editors was also appointed to further simplify the editing procedure and attain best results for the readers.

Apart from the editorial board, the designing team has also invested a significant amount of their time in understanding the subject and creating the most relevant covers. They scrutinized every image to scout for the most suitable representation of the subject and create an appropriate cover for the book.

The publishing team has been an ardent support to the editorial, designing and production team. Their endless efforts to recruit the best for this project, has resulted in the accomplishment of this book. They are a veteran in the field of academics and their pool of knowledge is as vast as their experience in printing. Their expertise and guidance has proved useful at every step. Their uncompromising quality standards have made this book an exceptional effort. Their encouragement from time to time has been an inspiration for everyone.

The publisher and the editorial board hope that this book will prove to be a valuable piece of knowledge for researchers, students, practitioners and scholars across the globe.

List of Contributors

Daniel I. Massé
Dairy and Swine Research and Development Centre, Agriculture and Agri-Food Canada, Sherbrooke, Quebec, J1M 0C8, Canada

Noori M. Cata Saady
Dairy and Swine Research and Development Centre, Agriculture and Agri-Food Canada, Sherbrooke, Quebec, J1M 0C8, Canada

Yan Gilbert
Dairy and Swine Research and Development Centre, Agriculture and Agri-Food Canada, Sherbrooke, Quebec, J1M 0C8, Canada

Bruno B. Chomel
Department of Population Health and Reproduction, School of Veterinary Medicine, University of California, Davis, CA 95616, USA

Elisabeth H. Ormandy
Animal Welfare Program, University of British Columbia, 2357 Main Mall, Vancouver, British Columbia, V6T 1Z4, Canada

Catherine A. Schuppli
Animal Welfare Program, University of British Columbia, 2357 Main Mall, Vancouver, British Columbia, V6T 1Z4, Canada

Nicole Fenwick
Canadian Council on Animal Care (CCAC), 190 O'Connor St., Suite 800, Ottawa, ON, K2P 2R3, Canada

Shannon E. G. Duffus
Canadian Council on Animal Care (CCAC), 190 O'Connor St., Suite 800, Ottawa, ON, K2P 2R3, Canada

Gilly Griffin
Canadian Council on Animal Care (CCAC), 190 O'Connor St., Suite 800, Ottawa, ON, K2P 2R3, Canada

Philip Bushby
College of Veterinary Medicine, Mississippi State University, P.O. Box 6001, Mississippi State, MS 39762, USA

Kimberly Woodruff
College of Veterinary Medicine, Mississippi State University, P.O. Box 6001, Mississippi State, MS 39762, USA

Jake Shivley
College of Veterinary Medicine, Mississippi State University, P.O. Box 6001, Mississippi State, MS 39762, USA

Graeme Coulson
Department of Zoology, The University of Melbourne, Parkville, VIC 3010, Australia Macropus Consulting, 105 Canning Street, Carlton, VIC 3053, Australia

Jemma K. Cripps
Department of Zoology, The University of Melbourne, Parkville, VIC 3010, Australia
Department of Environment and Primary Industries, Cnr. Midland Highway and Taylor Street, Epsom, VIC 3554, Australia

Michelle E. Wilson
Department of Zoology, The University of Melbourne, Parkville, VIC 3010, Australia
Wilson Environmental, 27 Ford Street, Brunswick, VIC 3056, Australia

Cristiano Fidani
Osservatorio Sismico "Andrea Bina", Borgo XX Giugno 74, 06121 Perugia, Italy
Central Italy Electromagnetic Network (CIEN), Via Fosso del Passo 6, 63847 San Procolo, Fermo, Italy

Friedemann Freund
Ames Research Center, National Aeronautics and Space Administration (NASA), Earth Science Division, Code SGE, Moffett Field, CA 94035, USA
Department of Physics, San Jose State University, San Jose, CA 95192, USA
Carl Sagan Center, SETI Institute, 189 Bernardo Ave., Mountain View, CA 94043, USA

Rachel Grant
Department of Life Sciences, Anglia Ruskin University, East Rd., Cambridge, CB1 1PT, UK

Printed in the USA
CPSIA information can be obtained
at www.ICGtesting.com
JSHW051447221024
72173JS00006B/1603

9 781682 860045